COPY[illegible]AIMER

Expert Consultants: Saleema Noon & Tara Johnson
Research: Yasaman Madanikia
Cover Design: New Media Graphix
ISBN: 978-0-9918904-4-6

Preface

If you haven't already done so, it's time to start having an open and honest dialogue with your children about sex and sexuality. Don't leave it up to the schools to address. Don't think *they're too young to know.* The truth is that the world is a different place to the one we grew up in and our children need our support and guidance to translate the constant sexualized messages they're getting from friends, the Internet and other media.

Not only does knowing about sexual health protect children from abuse, it also helps them learn about physical and behavioural boundaries, family values, gender identity, self-esteem, body image, how to interact with people, how to express themselves as individuals and more...

We know discussing sexuality with your children isn't easy or comfortable, but it can be done! We've consulted with experts, reviewed the literature extensively and distilled it into easy to read, manageable pieces along with talking points on how to **Start the Conversation** with your child. We're committed to helping you, make those tough conversations easy so that you in turn can help your children stay healthy and safe.

While in their Preschool years, a child's immediate family is their biggest influence, in their Primary years, children start going to school, seeing new things and meeting new people. Consequently, they're exposed to more outside influences and suddenly they start to question everything!

Sex Education: Curiosity Is Getting Complicated! Builds on the foundation laid in *Sex Education: It's More Than Learning About How Babies Are Made!* and takes a more detailed look into what children aged 6-8 want and need to know, from questions on puberty and multiple births to gender identity, bullying and sexual diversity.

Table of Contents

What You Should Know

Sexual dialogue is important because it gives your child the foundation to achieve health, respect and safety in their future relationships and protects them from sexual abuse. In fact, studies show that children who have been taught about sexuality from reliable adults wait longer to engage in sex, have fewer partners, and experience less incidences of teenage pregnancy and STI's.

Sex Education: Curiosity Is Getting Complicated! outlines the information that you should convey to your child as they grow through the ages of 6 to 8. It includes strategies for answering questions, and resources to assist their implementation.

What can you expect from children ages 6-8?

Independence

- *preferring to socialize with their own gender*
- *referencing external sources for answer to questions*
- *touching their genitals for pleasure or comfort*
- *same-gender sexual exploration*
- *body proprietorship manifesting as shyness and modesty*
- *owning the right to say NO*

What do children ages 6-8 need?

Context

- *sexual dialogue is important*
- *facts should not be confused with knowledge*
- *knowledge ensures health, respect, and safety in future relationships*
- *knowledge makes targeting by predators less likely*
- *sex is more than reproduction*
- *boundaries exist and should be respected*
- *bodies are private and should be respected*
- *understanding puberty*
- *understanding diversity*
- *understanding gender role stereotypes*

An Important Note!

Every child develops at their own rate, some earlier or later then others. No two children are exactly alike, each has their own personality and an approach that works for one, may not necessarily work for another. While these modules are designed as a support tool for the important discussions you'll have with your child, they are NOT rulebooks. Children don't always fit exactly into these age categories and the responsibility lies with you to gauge your child's emotional, mental and physical development in order to provide them with the correct information at the right time.

If you've read *Sex Education: It's More Than Learning About How Babies Are Made!* parts of this book may seem familiar. We hope you'll understand that we've kept some of the material the similar (but more age appropriate) for the benefit of those parents who don't have younger children and may not have had the opportunity to cover the essentials with their child.

Breaking The Ice

In this age group, kids' perceptions of the world start changing as the new perspectives they develop are predicated on rules, logic, and facts. Whether through school or media, their circle of influence is growing beyond the immediate family, which prompts many new questions as they attempt to rationalize their ever-expanding world.

Don't confuse facts with knowledge! Kids need context.

As illustrated, human sexuality is complex and extends well beyond the ins and outs of reproduction and sexual intercourse.

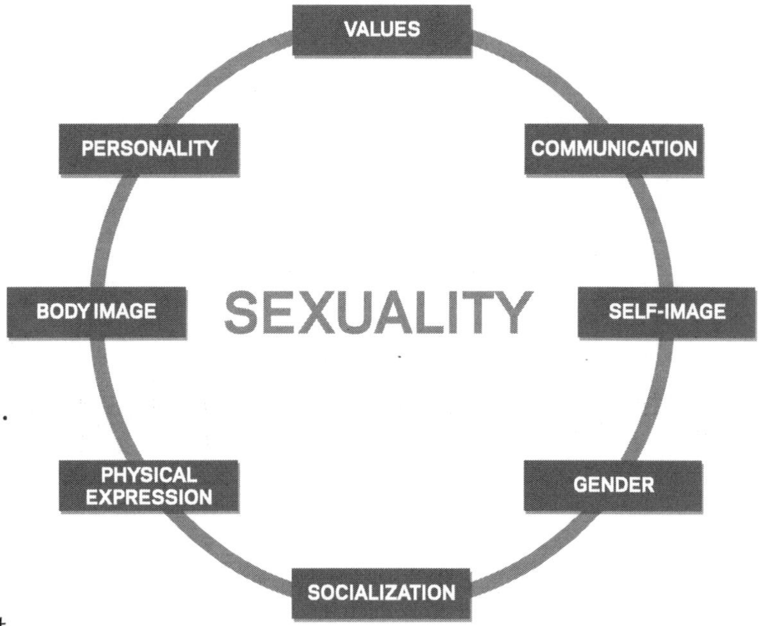

Where to begin

If your child is asking sex-oriented questions, it's a pretty clear indication that they're ready for the answers. Take this as a compliment! It means they trust you as a credible source of information. Now it's up to you to create a safe environment for their curiosity.

Don't avoid these conversations or leave it until your child starts asking questions or enters school. It's not the job of the educational system, the media, or peers to educate your kid! The responsibility lies with you to ensure that your child has a healthy, comprehensive sexual education. Some things are far too important to be left to chance or unreliable sources.

Don't feel badly if you're initially uncomfortable having these conversations. After all, most of us weren't raised in homes that encouraged open sexual dialogue.

When your child asks you a tough question, why not respond with a probing question of your own:

- *What do you think?*
- *Where did you hear that?*

- *Why are you asking?*
- *Tell me more...*

This allows you to find out where the question is coming from and clarify exactly what your child wants to know. It also buys you time to phrase a thoughtful, appropriate response! Even if you can't muster an immediate answer, make sure that you reinforce how happy you are that they asked the question. Let them know that you need some time to decide how best to answer. Don't make this a more challenging job than it needs to be! Take a deep breath, collect your thoughts, and re-approach the conversation when you're ready.
Don't change the subject or tell them that they're too young to know. Try not to giggle or show discomfort or annoyance either! This will only make them look elsewhere for information.

Timing and location are everything!

There's no perfect moment to discuss sexuality with your child but sometimes, hard conversations become easier when you have them in an appropriate environment like at bedtime, in the bedroom. While the subject is an important one, there's no need to get too serious! Games make marvellous teaching aides, play *Scientist*, for instance, and research the answers to their questions together!

How much information is enough?

Your child will let you know, as they'll change the subject or walk away when they've had enough. Information can't hurt them, but it CAN protect them.

Strategies

It helps to identify strategies that can assist you in starting natural, unforced conversations with your child. Take their personality into account, every child processes information differently. Many kid's books, Apps and movies provide ready-made scripts that explain concepts and answer questions. When you're engaging in these activities with your child, embrace open-ended, supportive comments like:

- *How do you think it happens?*
- *What do you think?*
- *What a great question!*

Validate their curiosity and keep the conversation going! As a parent, you need to take the lead on conversations about sexual health. Some children never ask questions because they're shy, embarrassed or are simply not that curious. If you remain silent too, they may see it as a sign that the topic is off limits.

Lead by example!

Kids mirror what they see. Modelling positive behaviours will have a positive impact on your child's perception of love, affection, conflict resolution, and their own bodies.
Your nonverbal cues like gestures, eye contact, and body language speak volumes about your perceptions of sex and sexuality. Talking to you child about sexual health doesn't have to be difficult, all you need to do is stick to the facts, keep it simple and use the right scientific terminology.

Be patient!

Answering and re-answering questions can be super frustrating but that's part of being a parent. Try to treat every scenario you encounter as a potential teaching moment and try to take these opportunities when they present themselves, sexuality is a dynamic process that continues to develop and change throughout life!
If your child's in a sex-ed class at school, it's important that you reinforce what they're being taught and are honest and age-appropriate in your conversations. Be proactive with your dialogue and open about the values and beliefs you hold. After all, you want to be your kid's primary source for sex education, right?
Remember, lessons like this often bear repeating and how you respond to your child's natural inquisitiveness will greatly influence their perceptions of their body and sexuality plus shape the tone of your future dialogue. Without it, questions may be answered by unsafe or unreliable sources.

Value this wonderful opportunity to be your child's primary influence!

BOTTOM LINE

- **Communication is the key to becoming an approachable parent! It's okay to be uncomfortable, starting the conversation is the most important thing. It becomes easier over time.**
- **As parents, it's up to you to start the conversation. Starting the conversation early sets you up as their go to source for information on sexual health.**
- **When your child asks you a question, clarify by responding with one of your own.**
- **When explaining sexual health to your child, stick to the facts, keep it simple and use the right scientific terminology.**
- **Model the behaviour you want your child to exhibit and commit to an honest, open dialogue about sexual health.**

In the next section...

Small things can make a big difference! Once you've started the conversation, it's important to teach your child what their body parts are and how they work because it can protect them from abuse.

The Bare Necessities

Kids in this age group are naturally curious about everything including *how* they compare physically to other children, *why* they're different and *how* their bodies work. Whereas before they were satisfied with the basics, now they want details!

What They Are

If you feel uncomfortable using the proper terms for body parts, start small and practice saying one word over and over. Once you're a little more comfortable, practice the scientific names for body parts with your child and try using them in conversation and you'll be amazed by how quickly it gets easier! We've all used jargon like *wee wee* and *vajayjay* to describe genitals but it's important that children know the scientific names for all their body parts, private or otherwise.

Explain that boys and girls have different private parts ...

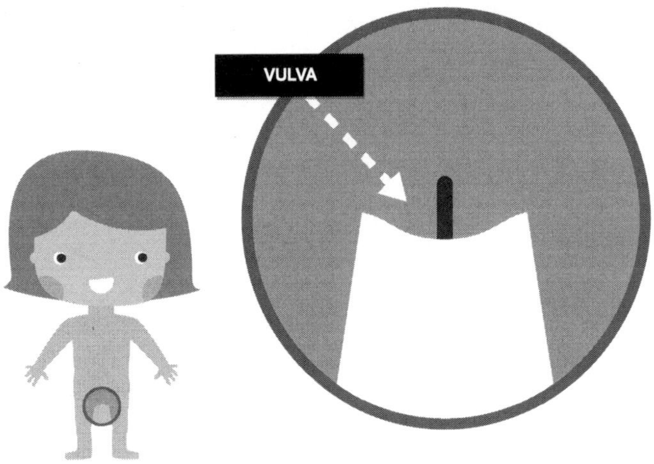

Girls have a vulva (labia) and boys have a penis.

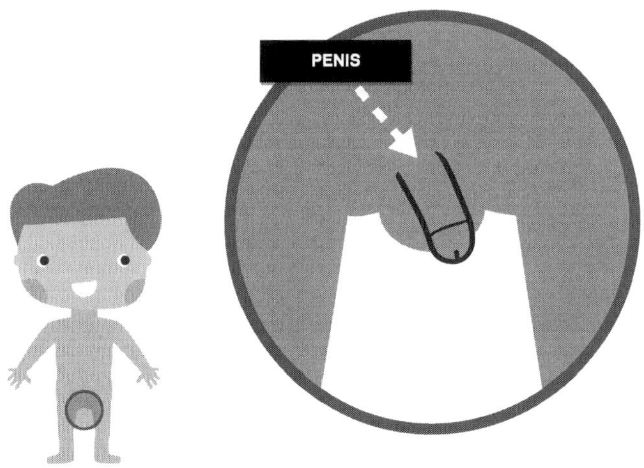

Girls also have:

- clitoris
- vagina
- anus
- urethra
- uterus
- ovaries

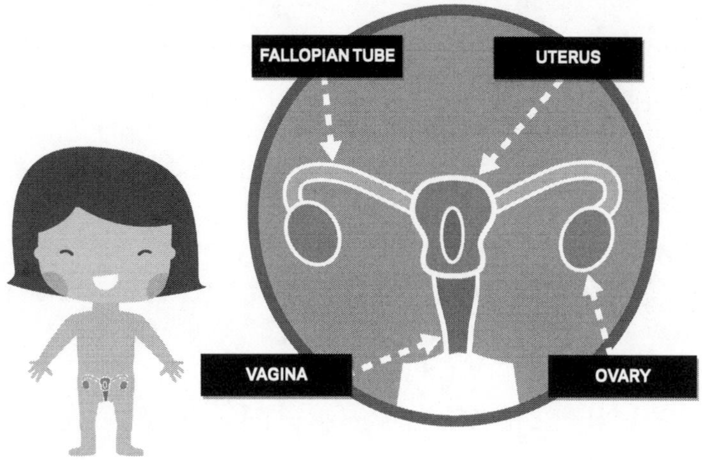

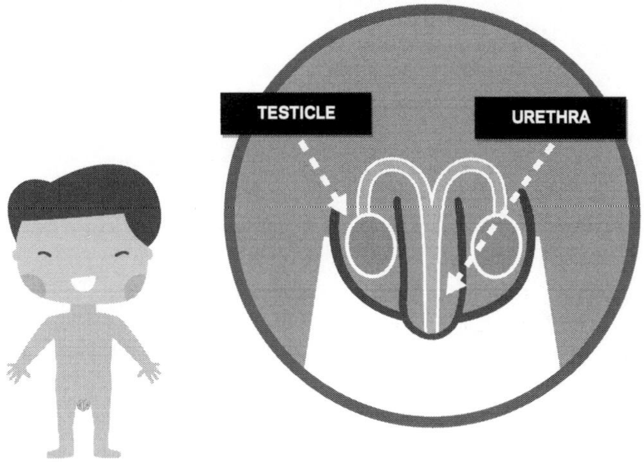

Boys also have:

- penis
- testicles
- scrotum
- urethra

Once kids start learning about these body parts, it's important that they understand that they're *private*. Collectively, *private parts* include:

- *genitals*
- *breasts*
- *mouth*

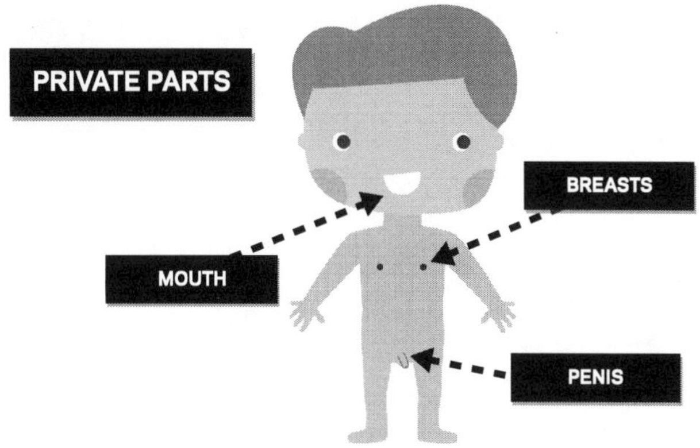

Bath time is a great opportunity to identify private parts in particular. Studies show that children who are informed about their bodies are more protected from sexual abuse, because they are more likely to report such behaviour to a trusted adult.

Conversely, a child who hasn't been taught ownership of their body is more susceptible to sexual predators because they haven't been taught to report inappropriate touching.

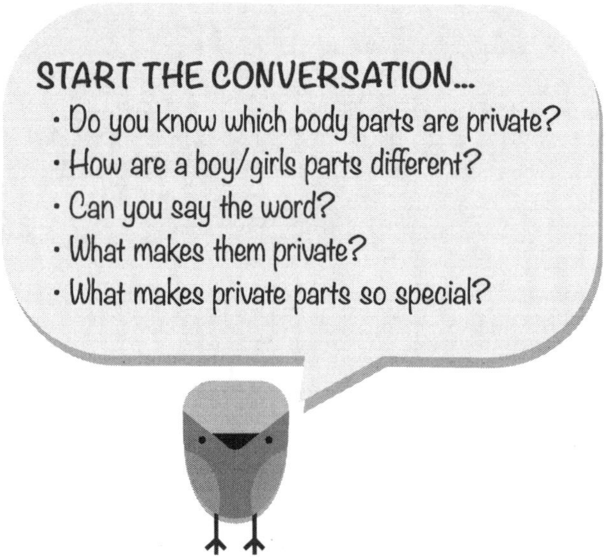
START THE CONVERSATION...
• Do you know which body parts are private?
• How are a boy/girls parts different?
• Can you say the word?
• What makes them private?
• What makes private parts so special?

How They Work

Children in this age group need to know the differences between their bodies and those of other children of BOTH sexes and more importantly, they need to understand *why* these differences exist.

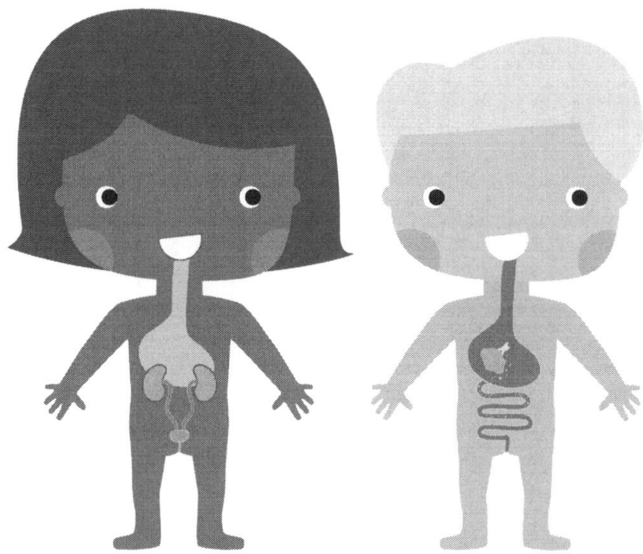

Boys are born with penises and girls are born with vulvas and vaginas. We're designed this way so that men and women can join like two puzzle pieces to make a baby. This happens when a man puts his penis in a woman's vagina and his sperm (seed) joins her ovum (egg).

(There's more on how babies are made in our chapter on *The Truth About Making Babies*).

Your child's education needs to include information about their digestive, urinary and reproductive systems as well. Why? Well, it's too easy to confuse the three. We've all heard kids use *tummy* synonymously with *womb*, we call sperm *a seed*, ovum *an egg*… and because children are very literal at this age, they might think that the mother ate the baby to get it in her tummy. If the baby is in her tummy, does she vomit or pooh to get the baby out of her tummy?
They should know that when baby's are born, they come out of their mother's body through her vagina and that the body produces waste from the liquids and solids that we consume, which leaves the body in two ways:

- *Urine (liquid waste) is produced in the kidneys and collected in the bladder. It exits the body through the urethra (located at the tip of the penis in boys and at the urethral opening between the vagina and clitoris in girls).*
- *Stool (solid waste) is produced after food travels from the mouth to the stomach, through the intestines. These unneeded materials exit the body through the anus.*

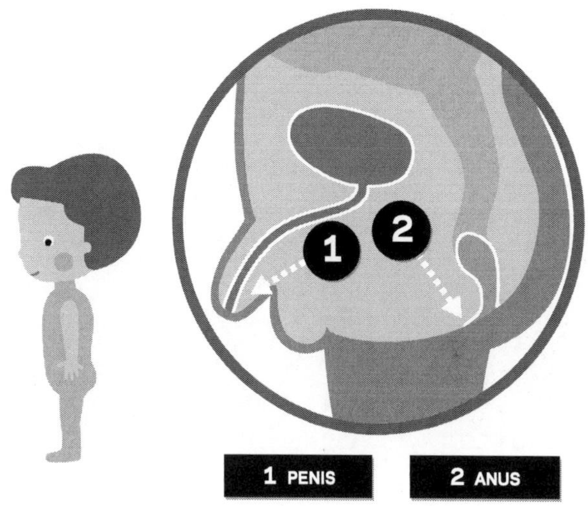

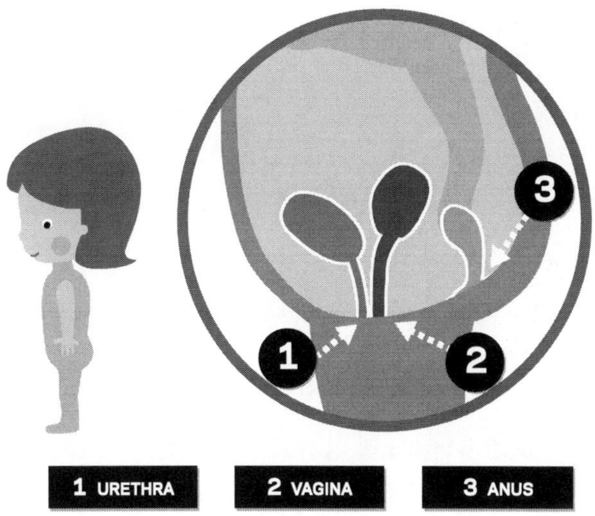

This is why boys only have 2 openings between their legs and girls have 3.

How do I explain practice erections?

Like any other muscle in the body, the penis needs exercise in order to remain healthy. Practice erections are the body's way of maintaining the health of the organ as it prepares for sexual activity later in life. Erections begin in the womb and are a normal, healthy part of male development.

Let your son know that when he has an erection, his penis is practicing to have a baby when he's older. Be aware of appropriate boundaries, though, as he may need to be reminded about privacy when engaging in self-stimulation!

START THE CONVERSATION ...

- Do you know why girls have an extra opening?
- What do you think?
- How do you think babies get in a mommy's womb?
- Do you know the difference between a tummy and a womb?
- Why do you think a boys penis goes up and down sometimes?
- Where do you think food goes after we put it in our mouths?
- How do you think babies get out of the mommy's womb?
- Where do you think urine (pee) comes from?
- Do you know where it comes out of the body?
- Do you know where it comes from?

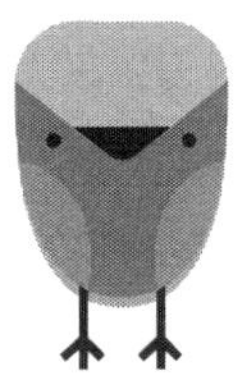

Keep It Clean!

If you haven't already, it's a good idea to have the genital hygiene chat! Don't assume that your kid knows how to wash properly, it's a skill that takes both direction and practice!

If neglected, smegma (a white, odorous substance) can collect under the skin of the penis and between the folds of the vulva. Show your child how to clean their private parts just like you would if you were teaching them to wash any other body part. When kids are comfortable

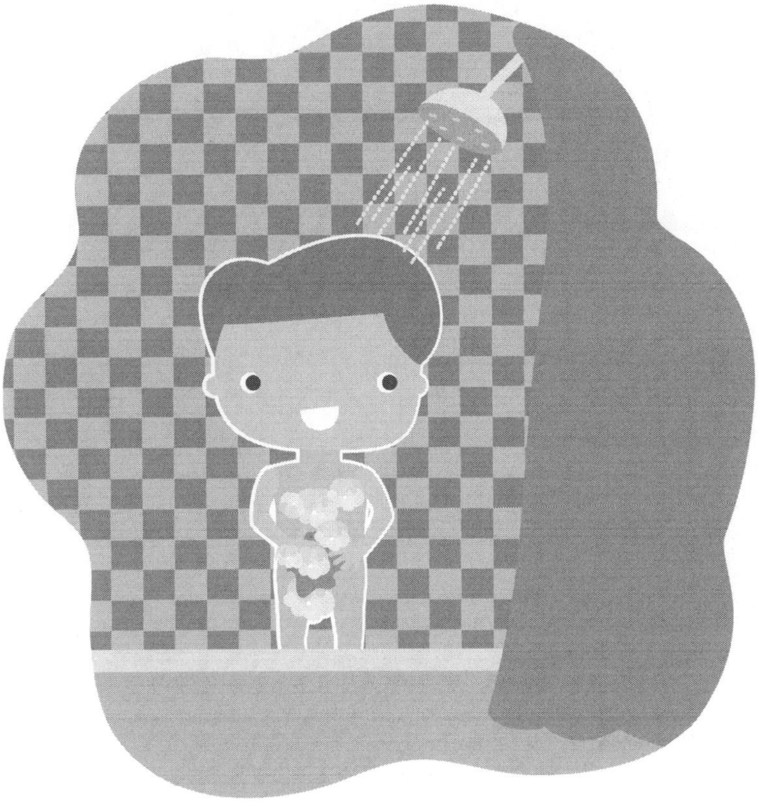

with this, they're equipped to recognize when something's wrong. Remember to teach your daughter to wipe down and away from the vulva, especially after a bowel movement, since stool can cause an infection if it enters the urethra. Advise your son to sleep naked or in loose underwear because testicles should be kept below body temperature.

Although it's rare, intense testicular or abdominal pain can be the result of something called testicular torsion, which happens when the testicles twist inside the scrotal sac. If this occurs, seek immediate medical attention.

START THE CONVERSATION ...

- Why do you think it's important to clean your private parts?
- Do you think it's a good idea for children to clean their private parts every day?

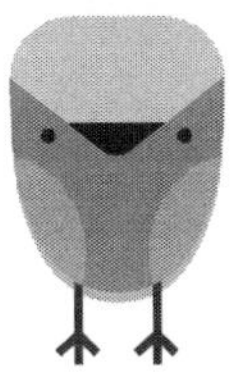

What's Wrong With My Penis?

Your son has probably noticed that his penis looks different or similar to other penises. He's likely compared his penis to his dad's, too and wondered why they look different. Reassure him that all penises are different but work exactly the same way. When a baby is born, some families decide to remove the foreskin surrounding the tip of the penis. Either way, this doesn't affect the health, cleanliness, or functionality of the penis.

Don't avoid the circumcision discussion! Ignorance can lead to anxiety and feelings of alienation.

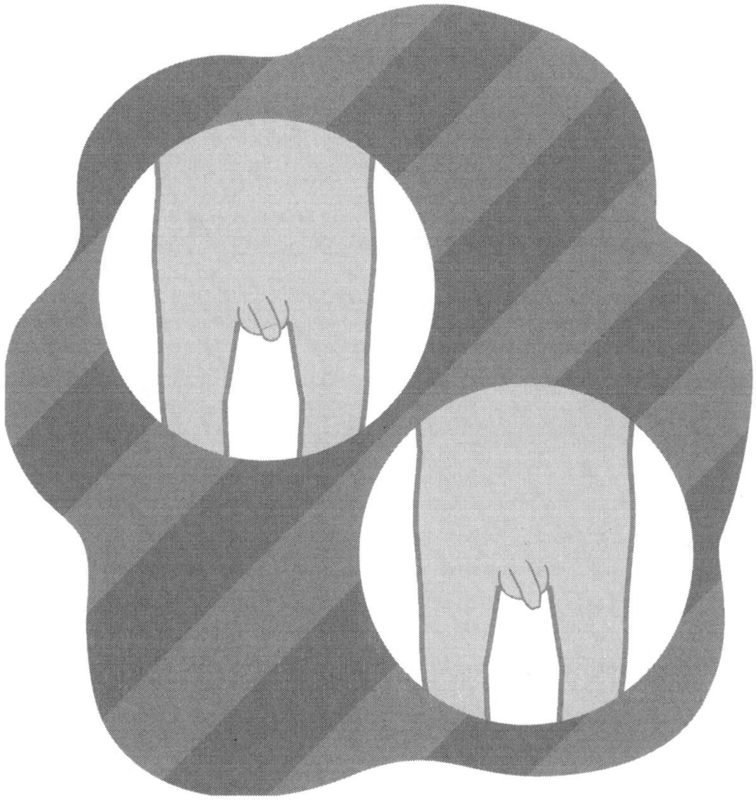

START THE CONVERSATION ...

- What do you think of your penis?
- Have you seen/noticed penises that look different to yours?
- How are they different to yours?

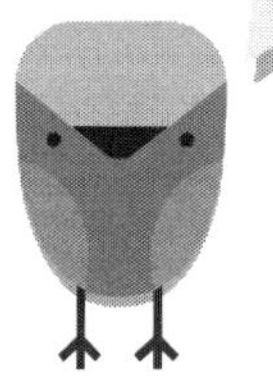

Poking Fun at Pooh!

Most kids this age are excessively preoccupied with *bathroom humour* and there's little that you as a parent can do about it. They use it as a means of creating dialogue about sexuality, biology, and boundaries and to make it worse, the behaviour is fuelled by the laughter, shock, or even anger it garners. How do you handle the onslaught of underwear quips, private part zingers and bodily function knock-knock jokes?

Stay Calm!

First, deal with the inappropriate elements of your kid's language, reminding them that they don't need to use nicknames to describe private parts. Secondly, contextualize their behaviour. Try to figure out if it's coming from a place of curiosity or a need for attention.

It doesn't hurt to review the correct terminology for reproductive organs and re-explain how pregnancy and reproduction occur. Bathroom humour can usually be preempted when the content of their jokes is demystified.

The peer-pressure to use colloquialisms can be overwhelming, especially for little boys. Most kids take some time to grow out of this stage so stay patient and don't be afraid to repeat yourself. And repeat yourself. And repeat yourself...

Try not to overreact! Your emotional response can actually serve to escalate the behaviour and attach misplaced value to the situation. Remember, they're just trying to make sense of their sexuality, privacy, and boundaries!

Soaking Sheets?

Waking up with urine-soaked pyjamas is super upsetting for any child. Bedwetting, which is common in kids ages six to eight, appears to be hereditary and can sometimes last into the teen years. If your son or daughter is consistently wetting the bed, it's probably because they're unable to wake themselves when their bladder's full. Barring extenuating causes, the problem will normally stop on its own.

Is your child suffering from sudden onset bedwetting? Several factors could be responsible:

- *urinary tract infections (UTIs)*
- *structural bladder problems*
- *extreme stress*
- *diabetes*
- *emotional/psychological trauma*

It's a good idea to rule out urinary tract infection first by checking to make sure that the urine

is clear, not cloudy or pink. If you suspect an infection, see the doctor immediately!
UTIs can be caused by a number of factors:

- *wiping toward the front instead of the back*
- *forgetting to wash hands after using the bathroom*
- *sexual abuse*

If your child experiences any of the following situations, there may be a health-related issue deserving of a doctor's attention:

- *starts wetting themselves during the day*
- *has to urinate frequently*
- *experiences swelling of the feet/ankles*
- *starts drinking more liquids than usual*
- *complains of a burning sensation/pain when urinating*
- *starts bedwetting after being consistently dry*
- *starts bedwetting after the age of seven*

While you're at the doctor's office, ask that your child's urine is tested for microbes. *E.coli* are responsible for most UTIs but testing positive for *Chlamydia* may indicate inappropriate touching.
If there's no specific cause for the bedwetting, reassure your child that they'll grow out of it. If you were a bed-wetter yourself, let them know. Empathy goes a long way! In the meantime, take a practical approach to the problem: avoid beverages with diuretic qualities, like sodas, coffee or tea. Little reminders about pre-bed time bathroom breaks are helpful too. If the condition is chronic (as often it can be) buy a waterproof mattress cover for the bed. Most importantly, remain patient, and remember to heap on the praise on dry nights!

START THE CONVERSATION ...

- You can tell me if anything is bothering you. Can we talk about it?
- How is everything at school?
- How do you feel when you wet the bed? Reassure and be empathetic.
- How is your body feeling?

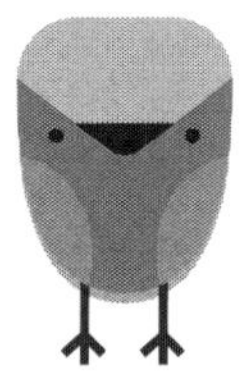

What's Going to Happen to Me?

Most kids of this age have been exposed to information about puberty, whether through family, friends, or media. This is why it's so important that they know the basics about puberty and how it changes their bodies. Bedtime's an ideal time to initiate these kinds of conversations, especially with kids who are less inclined to do the asking.

The process of puberty starts as early as age 8, continuing until approximately age 18. Although the changes are (for the most part) the same for each gender, every child develops a little bit differently.

Explain that puberty is just the body's way of preparing for reproduction. During this time, girls' bodies grow taller, broader and heavier, their breasts begin to develop, and hair starts to grow under their arms and on their pubis. They also begin producing vaginal discharge (smegma) and begin to sweat more.

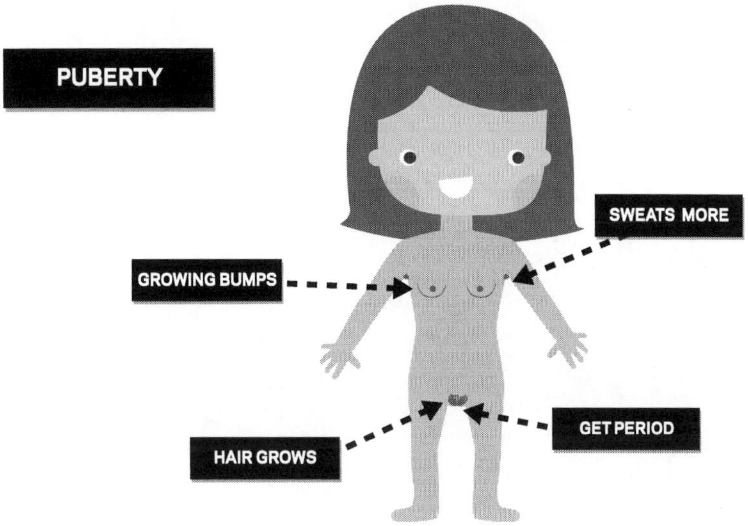

Girls can experience their first period or *menarche* when they are as young as eight, although the average age is closer to 12 or 13. Make sure your daughter understands menstruation and what to expect during this natural, healthy process! Don't skip this conversation or say I'll tell you when you're older. The visibility of feminine products makes this one of the easiest teachable moments to have and having a period when you don't know what it is can be frightening to a child! (We'll elaborate on menstruation in the *It's Only A Period!* chapter later).

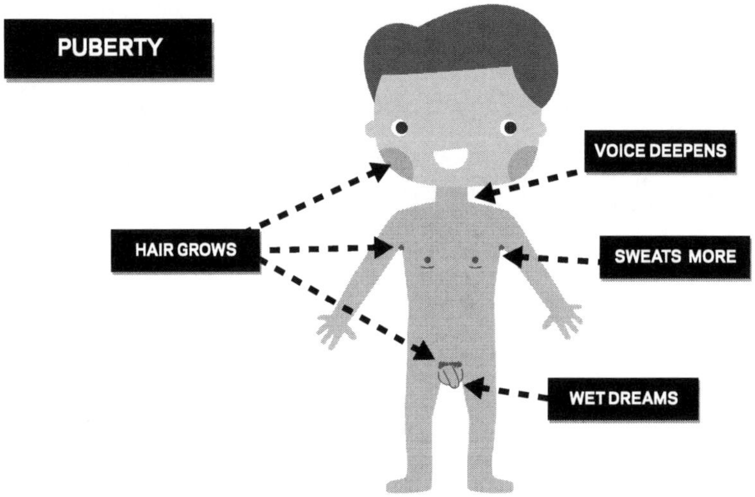

When boys begin puberty, their bodies grow taller and wider, their voices becomes deeper, they experience wet dreams (nocturnal emissions) and hair starts to grow under their arms and on their pubis. They also begin to sweat more.

START THE CONVERSATION ...

- What do you think puberty means?
- How do you think your body is different to an older girl/boy?
- Have you heard anything about puberty?
- Do you know what happens to a girl during puberty?
- Do you know what happens to a boy during puberty?
- When do you think puberty happens?
- Who do you think puberty happens to?
- What does puberty mean to you?

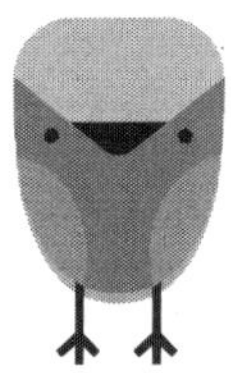

BOTTOM LINE:

- **When explaining body parts and functions, use the proper scientific words.**
- **Explain to your child that girls have three openings between their legs and boys have two.**
- **Don't forget to teach your child about the parts and functions of the opposite sex.**
- **Learning how to clean genitals is a learned skill that needs to be taught for reasons of hygiene and for children to recognize if something is wrong with them.**
- **Remember to be patient and not to overreact if children in this age group seem preoccupied with bathroom humour.**
- **Puberty can start in children as young as 8. Don't skip the conversation, preparing children in advance will make them better equipped with the changes their bodies will go through.**

In the next section....

In addition to knowing the names and functions of their private parts, children need to learn their rights and identify their boundaries in order to stay safe and healthy

Where to Draw the Line

For children in this age group, exploration is their way of discovering their bodies' behavioural and physical boundaries in relation to world they live in. Your role is to help your child recognize *what* is appropriate, understand *why*, and identify *where* the limits lay.

I'm My Own Body Boss

Teach your child to be their own body boss!

Make sure your child can identify their own private parts *(mouth, breast, genitals)* as well as the private parts of the opposite sex, using a picture or toy to help illustrate the differences. Reinforce boundaries. Not only does your child need to understand the names and functions of their private parts. They need learn their rights and identify their boundaries as well.
Give examples of appropriate behaviour (i.e. parents changing diapers, dentists looking in mouths) and inappropriate behaviour (i.e. unwanted kisses, play involving touching of genitals).

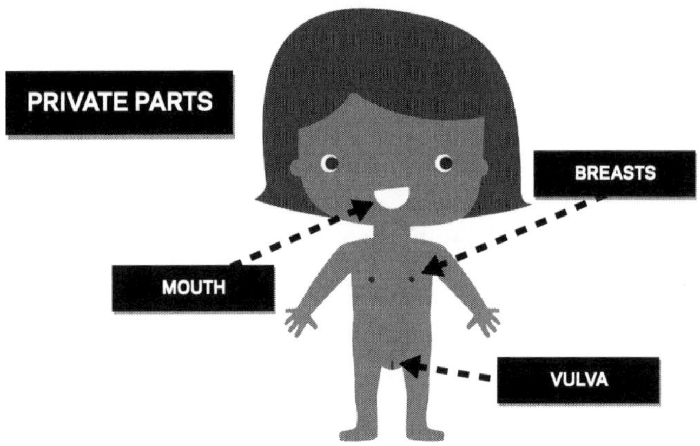

Carefully explain that it's inappropriate for anyone to touch or kiss their private parts or for them to touch or kiss the private parts of others. This includes friends, siblings, family, teachers, coaches, and neighbours. It's only appropriate for parents to clean a child's genitals or a doctor to examine them (providing a parent is present). Make sure they understand that if anyone tells them this behaviour is *okay* or to *keep it a secret*, that it's wrong. They have the right to say NO and must let you (or a trusted adult) know immediately if this happens. Remind your child that if the person they report to doesn't believe or help them immediately, they must report to someone else and keep reporting until someone helps them.
Be careful not to force your child to kiss or hug someone whom they don't want to because it

sends mixed messages and teaches them to ignore their instincts. A forced hug or kiss is disrespectful to the child. Instead, why not ask *Does Aunt Nancy get a hug today?* This empowers the child to make the decision. If it's a no hugs day, high fives and waves can take their place. Forcing a child to kiss someone against their will is asking them to use their mouth (a private part) against their will.

START THE CONVERSATION ...

- Do you know/remember what makes private parts so special?
- What does a good touch feel like? A hug from mom and dad?
- When is it okay for someone to touch another person? (E.g. Doctor's appointment or a mom changing a baby's diaper).
- Tell me about when you don't want to say hi to someone with a kiss and hug?
- How does that make you feel? Can you say why?
- What could you do instead of a hug or kiss?
- What can you say if you don't want to hug or kiss someone?
- It's important you listen to what your body says, hi fives or handshakes are good too.
- What do you think if an adult wants to touch a child?
- What do you think you should do if someone touches you in your private parts?

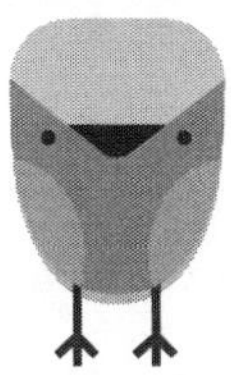

Safety: What Every Parent Needs to Know!

Knowledge is protection!

The body boss and body boundaries lessons are important because they boost awareness, build confidence and most importantly, offer protection. As parents, our worst fear is having our child targeted by predators. Let's face it, the topic of sexual abuse is a sensitive one but when the stats are so staggering (1 out of 4 girls and 1 out of 6 boys will be sexually abused by age 18) it's not a topic that can be ignored. Keep in mind that 90-percent of those who abuse children are in and around the family, not strangers lurking in the sidelines. Take the following information to heart.

Regardless of who's committing the abuse, there are commonalities among all perpetrators:

Many perpetrators utilize what experts call the *grooming process.* Grooming (which usually starts well in advance of the act of abuse) is a gradual process that involves gaining the trust of both the child and their family. This is done to develop trust and lower the child's inhibitions in preparation for sexual abuse. Children who know and trust an offender are much less likely to report the abuse. Predators prefer getting close to their victim's family because their proximity makes the child's story seem less believable if the abuse happens to be reported.

The labels vary, but most sexual abuse will involve the following 6 steps:

1. **Targeting the child**
2. **Gaining their trust**
3. **Filling a special need**
4. **Isolating the child from their peers**
5. **Sexualising the relationship, and finally**
6. **Maintaining control over the child.**

Most sexual offenders are quite calculating with their attention and affection and know exactly how to balance the way that they interact with the child publicly and privately to avoid detection. Children who are being groomed by a predator will often idealize the offender, who seduces them into believing that they share a *special* relationship. This often leads to victims becoming willing participants in their own abuse.
When the trust of the child is gained, the abuser will start to desensitize the child to sexualising the relationship and make them believe that this is normal behaviour. Sexual offenders desensitize a child to the sexualising process by crossing the line bit by bit over time (eg. walking in when they're dressing).

Once an offender has sexualised a relationship with a child, it's easier to manipulate the child's physical response, which in turn reinforces the child's emotional attachment. Sexually abused children don't realize that their physical response to stimulation is beyond their control, which leads to feelings of guilt.

The abuser will leverage this in order to manipulate the child into thinking that the abuse is their fault. Sexual offenders keep children in an abusive relationship by using lack of self-esteem, guilt and emotional vulnerability.
Abused children can become more afraid of the consequences of telling (isolation, humiliation) than suffering the ongoing abuse.

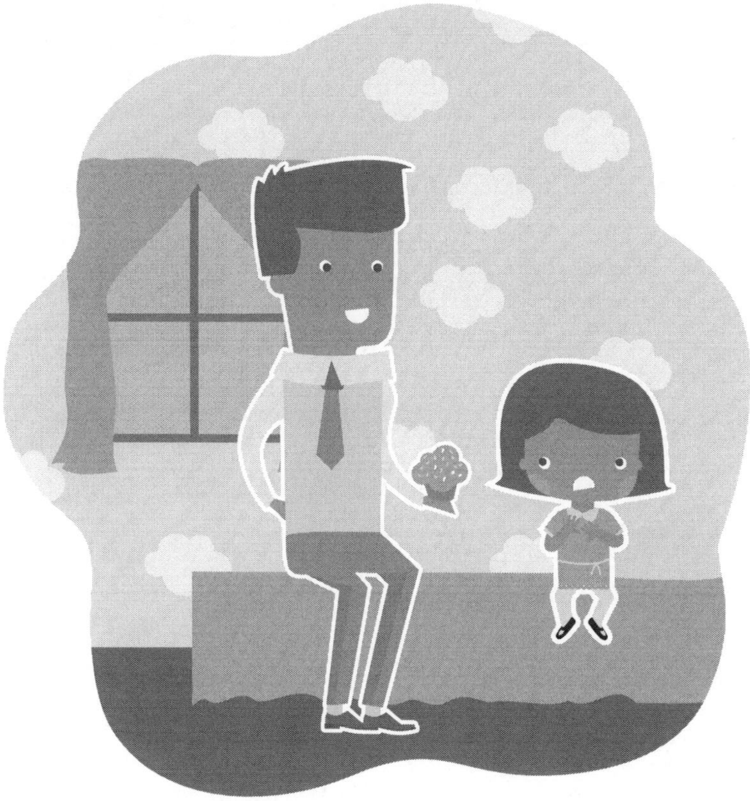

ALWAYS believe the child!

7 Things to look out for:

- Adults that seem to give more attention to children than other adults.
- Child molesters will seek out places children frequent (parks, sports grounds, shopping malls etc)
- Adults who like to be in physical contact with children a lot. i.e., tickling, wrestling and have children sit on their lap.
- Adults who your child idealizes for reasons you DO NOT understand.
- An adult who is always finding reasons to be around and is always offering to watch the children.
- An adult in or around the family showing a child undue attention, giving them gifts or money for no apparent reason.
- Adults that try to make opportunities (babysitting, coaching, trips, sleepovers) to spend time alone with your child.

11 Signs of abuse:

- Is the child afraid of a family member or another adult? Investigate!
- Is the child behaving in a sexual manner that is not age appropriate?

- Is the child exhibiting behaviour that is not developmentally appropriate? Ask questions and investigate.
- Is there blood in the child's underwear or do they have chronic bladder infections?
- Does the child act secretive about the unexplained acquisition of gifts / toys?
- Do they masturbate excessively? It may be innocent but it's worth looking into.
- The child tells you that they have a *secret* and *can't tell.*
- Regressive behaviour such as thumb sucking.
- The child acting out sexually with toys or inserting foreign objects into their vagina or anus.
- Night terrors and soiling the bed after being potty trained. Many children can demonstrate this for various reasons. It's worth looking at closer if it becomes more common.
- Unexplained behaviour such as incessantly crying and clinginess for no reason. Ask questions and investigate.

START THE CONVERSATION ...

- Explain to your child that some adults have touching problems and they touch children's private parts when they're not supposed to. These people are sick and need help. Ask
- Do you know anyone with a touching problem?
- What is an example of a good secret? A bad secret?
- What do you think about when touching is a secret?
- What do you think about adult and children touching or kissing each other's private parts?
- What should you do if someone asks you to touch someone else's private parts?

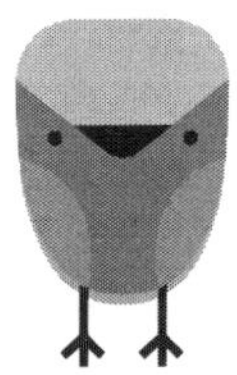

Tips on Teaching Privacy and Respect

Children have a natural tendency to explore boundaries, referencing their parents for guidance on where the limits lay. Your kid may begin talking non-discriminately about private parts or self-stimulation, or may even ask strangers about sex-related issues.

The best way to drive home a sense of privacy is by describing the private parts and reviewing behaviours that are appropriate versus ones that aren't.

Tell them that you're happy they can express themselves using the correct scientific names for body parts and reinforce that their bodies are indeed something to be proud of. Just makes sure you follow it up with a little reminder that the best place for these discussions is in the privacy of the home.

Private parts include the mouth plus anything that the swimsuit covers (including everything between their legs, from the lower back to their navel). It's not appropriate to show or discuss private parts in public because private means that they are not for other people to see, touch, or kiss.

Remind your child that when they're changing, taking a shower or using the bathroom, they should do so with the door closed and no one should come into the room without their permission.

START THE CONVERSATION ...

- What makes you happy about your body? Reinforce the positive.
- Why are private parts private? Reinforce that they are special to the person that owns them.
- Do you think its proper to discuss private parts with others outside the home? Why?
- When we talk about private parts it's important we don't share that information with other people. Do you know why?

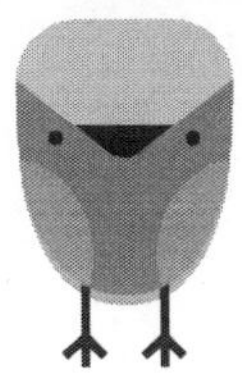

Exploration and Touching

Don't be surprised if your kid is playing with their genitals! From an early age, children are naturally curious about how their bodies work and *Self-Stimulation* or *Masturbation* (i.e. touching one's body for sexual pleasure) is perfectly normal, healthy, exploratory behaviour that kids do to feel pleasure, experience comfort, or sometimes just out of curiosity and boredom. Your daughter may comment that she feels *ticklish* or *funny down there*. Your son may mention that his *penis is standing up.* This is due simply to the rush of blood to the genitalia.

While normal and healthy, children often touch themselves in public, so it's important to remind them that their genitals are private and they shouldn't touch them in front of other people.

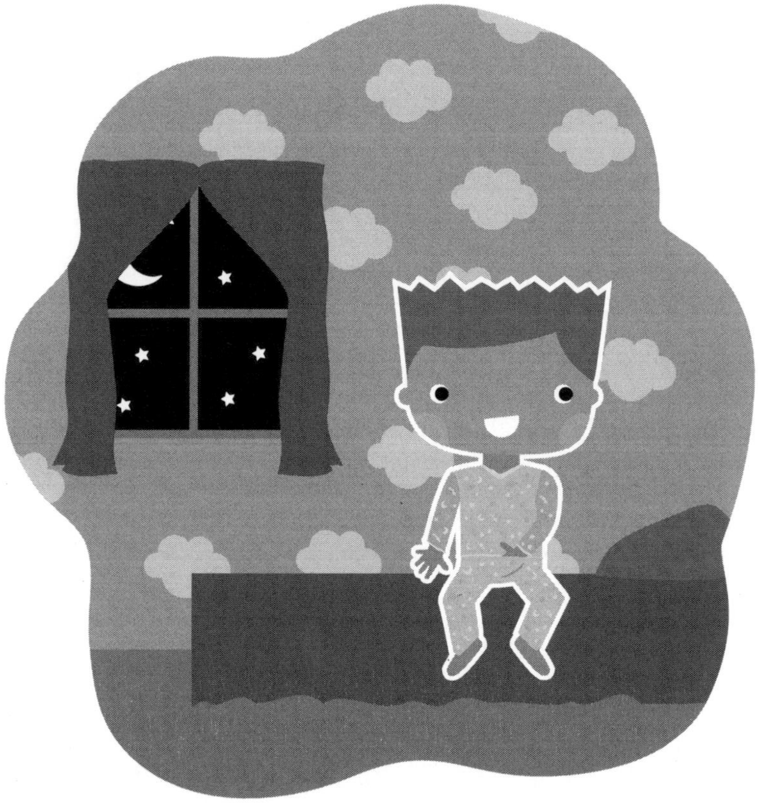

Playing Doctor

So you've discovered your child and another child examining each other's genitals…

Children's tendency to *play doctor* or *house* is prompted by the need to physically compare themselves with other kids, and that includes both sexes. This is actually pretty common among kids in the same age group. If however, an older kid is involved, the behaviour needs to be stopped immediately!

Most of the time, playing doctor comes from a place of natural curiosity and requires nothing more than re-direction to a more appropriate activity but be observant! Initial reactions speak volumes about whether or not your kid understands the inappropriateness of their behaviour. Calmly ask little Dr. Curious to get dressed, reminding them that private parts are special and need to be kept private from other people. Later, initiate a more detailed conversation in which you identify the private parts (*mouth, breasts, genitals)* by their scientific names and answer any questions that arise from the discussion.

The Other Kid

If you suspect that the other child may have influenced yours to engage in sexual play, be sure to investigate!

Discuss the incident with the other child's parents using a neutral, non-accusatory tone. Respect their boundaries, too! Whatever's occurred, it's for them to decide how to address the situation with their child. If you have to, place boundaries on your child's involvement with the playmate in question and monitor future play-dates carefully until you feel comfortable. Of course, the easiest way to preempt this behaviour is to instate an open door policy at home and on play-dates.

Inappropriate Touching at Home

Since some kids are more sensual than others, parents will invariably encounter varying degrees of inappropriateness.

Some kids may grab parents' / siblings' breasts / genitals. Some may like it when others touch their private parts. Your child needs to respect the privacy of others as well as their own, which

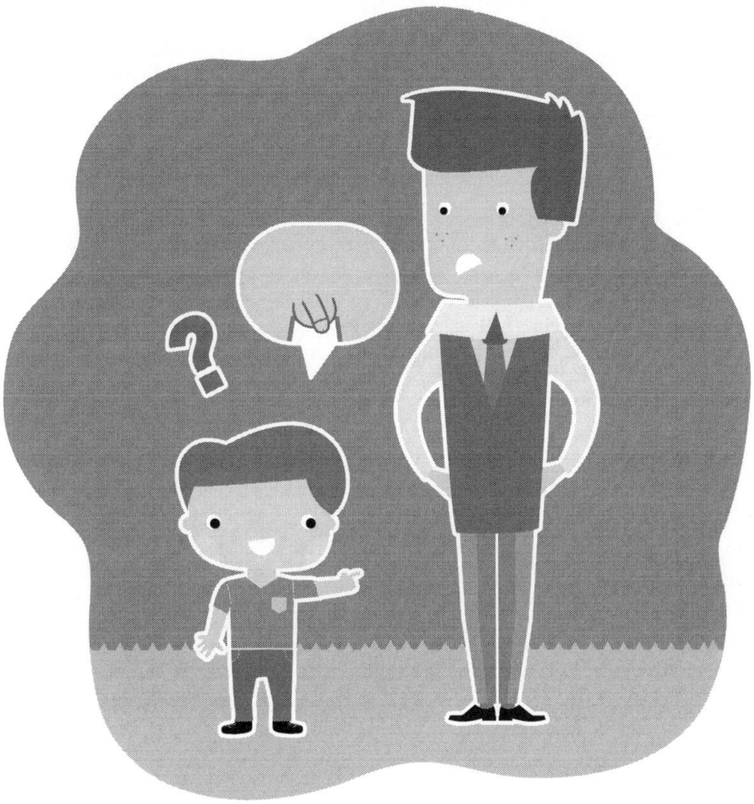

is why it's so important to reinforce boundaries whenever opportunities arise.

If your kid asks you to touch their genitals or vice-versa, don't be afraid to express your boundaries. Be sure your child knows where and what their private parts are. If they attempt to explore their body (or someone else's) in public, immediately remind them that this isn't appropriate. Private parts are very special to the person who owns them and it's not appropriate to grab other people's genitals or breasts. Acknowledge that it's fine for them to touch themselves providing they're alone.

When your child engages in inappropriate touching, don't use dismissive phrases such as:

- *It's just a phase*
- *They'll grow out of it*
- *It's just kids being kids*

If your kid's curiosity becomes obsessive, initiate an honest discussion, reminding them to tell you if any inappropriate behaviour occurs so that you can keep them safe.

START THE CONVERSATION ...

- Do you know what private/public means?
- Where is it appropriate to touch yourself (Bedroom/bathroom)?
- Do you know what private is/means?
- I know it feels good when you touch yourself but do you know where it is appropriate to do so?
- Why do you think it's important to keep it private?
- I understand you're curious about how other people bodies look, like (insert child's name). What interests you? Can you share with me what you want to know? It's not appropriate to share our own or touch other people's private parts, because they are special to the person that owns them. Please come to me and I'll help you with what you want to know.

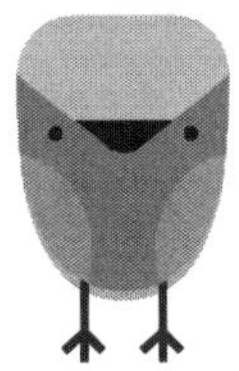

Nakedness

Time has a way of redefining boundaries. Be verbal if you begin feeling uncomfortable with your kid's nudity. Explain to them that they're getting too grown up to share your bath/walk around naked. Remind them that while there's absolutely nothing wrong with nudity, there comes an age when they must respect their privacy and that of others.

Too often with parents, it's a case of *Do as I say, not as I do.* Many mums and dads don't realize when their own behaviour is inappropriate. It may have been fine to be naked around your child when they were younger but with age they'll often grow uncomfortable with your nudity, too.

Pay attention to nonverbal cues! Your child may not want to hurt your feelings by verbalizing their discomfort at your nakedness. If they begin closing doors when they bathe or undress, it's a good indication that you should do likewise. Reassure them that it's okay to feel private about their bodies and that you respect their need for privacy. As long as both child and parent are verbal with their comfort levels and boundaries, everyone's privacy will be respected, however it evolves.

START THE CONVERSATION ...

- Are you feeling like you need more privacy to get dressed? We respect that.
- Would you like me/mom/dad to do the same?
- You're getting older and it's okay to feel more private. What would you like the house rules on boundaries, like nakedness, to be?

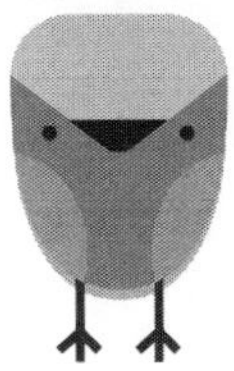

Sex Toys

Sometimes, children accidentally find sex toys around the house, causing unexpected (and often embarrassing) lines of questioning.

Keeping your sex toys out of reach or safely locked away is the easiest way to avoid this situation but nothing's a guarantee and no one's perfect. If this happens to you, calmly let your child know that what they've found is a special toy some adults like use when they have sex. In most cases, a simple answer will satisfy their curiosity. Stick to the facts and don't make a fuss! Kids will take their cue from you when it comes to comfort levels. A poor response from you will just attach negative/shameful connotations to something innocent and healthy.

START THE CONVERSATION ...

- What did you see? What do you think it's used for?
- What questions do you have?

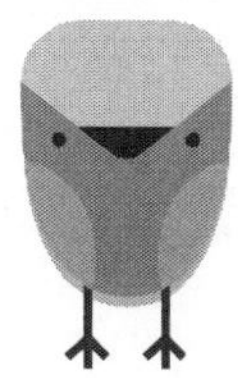

Walk-ins

Few things are more disturbing to hear coming from the foot of the bed than the question, *What are you doing?* But let's face it, walk-ins happen.

If you think you'll never forget the moment your kid discovered you and your partner in the throes of hot sex, imagine how they feel. Don't flub your lines! Your response will not only influence their perceptions of sexuality but also shape the tone of your future dialogue.

Politely ask your kid to leave the room and tell them you'll be with them momentarily. During the chat, explain that you and your partner were having some private time together and that no one was being hurt, despite how it may have appeared. Remind them that adults engage in these sorts of activities to show love and affection for one another.

If they want more information on reproduction, now's a good time to get into the basic biology of the whole thing, if you haven't already.

Don't forget to address the privacy issue! If your bedroom door was open, take responsibility for your carelessness. If it wasn't, remind them that it's polite to knock and wait for a response before entering certain rooms.

START THE CONVERSATION ...

- What did you see? What do you think was happening?
- What questions do you have?
- Do you think there should be rules about our closed door? I would ask you to knock next time you see our door closed. Are you okay with that?
- Did that scare you? There is nothing to be scared about. We were loving each other in a special way that adults do when they love each other.

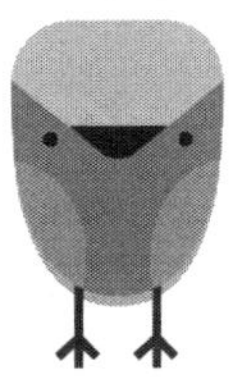

The Rules of Engagement

Most parents are familiar with stranger danger. The idea that individuals are lurking in the shadows waiting to snatch your child the minute you turn around is every parent's worst nightmare. Society has become hypersensitive to this notion but statistically only a small percentage of children are harmed by strangers.

90% of abuse is committed by someone the family knows and 50% of abusers are family members.

Nevertheless, vigilance and education are the best ways to protect your child and make them aware of their own safety. It's impossible to anticipate every situation that your child may encounter but there are still ways you can help them avoid potentially dangerous situations. **What is a stranger? A stranger is someone that you and your child don't know.** Teach your child to stay close in busy environments such as playgrounds, fairs, parks, and shopping malls and let them know it's imperative that they're always within visual range. Provide strategies and procedures to implement if they get lost. If they're in a mall or a built-up area, tell them to approach a shopkeeper and report that they're lost. If they're outdoors or away from developed areas, tell them to stay put. When you realize your child is lost, report it immediately to security personnel or a staff member as most buildings have a protocol for these situations.

Have your child memorize their address and phone number and teach them how to use 911 (your regional emergency number) in the event of an emergency. Repetitively reinforce that it's never appropriate to speak to strangers beyond acceptable polite conversation.

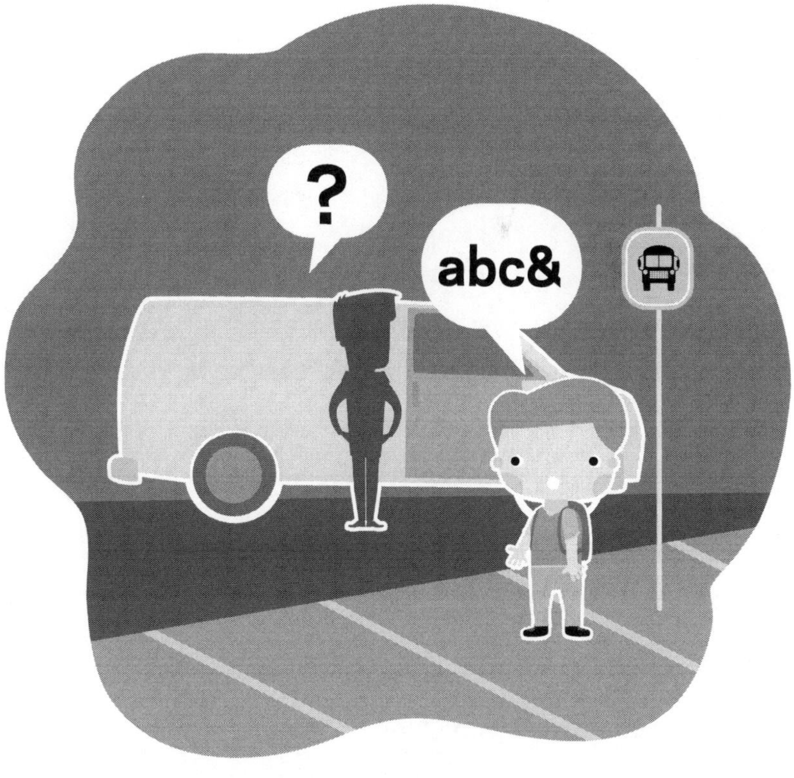

Remind them to seek the help of a trusted adult if they're lost or need help and teach them to trust their instincts. Provide them with examples of how a stranger might attempt to get their attention (e.g. candy, puppies, toys). Some ploys are more nefarious.

Some strangers may ask for their help or say that they're friends with their parents. Teach your child to NEVER go anywhere with a stranger. Give them a codeword or phrase that only you or someone you trust would know, instructing them to NEVER go anywhere with someone who doesn't know it.

Paranoia

Conversely, it's important not to instil paranoia. It's critical that they understand each of these situations and know not to judge a book by its cover. Remind your child that strangers can also be kind, friendly and helpful. It's not about being afraid of strangers. It's about knowing the rules for interacting with them. Arming your child with the right tools will help them remain safe and empower them to say NO when strangers attempt to engage them.

START THE CONVERSATION ...

- What is a stranger? What do they look like?
- Can you think of different types of trusted adults?
- If a stranger was knocking on the door, would you answer?
- If you are lost, who is a trusted adult you could go to in public? Police officer?
- If you are lost would you know what to do?
- Can you tell me other people who wear a uniform who aren't police officers?
- Can you think of a special (code) word that we could have together?
- What should you do/say if the stranger doesn't know the code word?
- Can you think of things the stranger might say if they don't know the code word to make you go with them?
- Do you think it's okay to say hello/goodbye to a stranger?
- When is it not okay to talk to a stranger?
- What do you say when that happens?
- Is it okay to accept gifts from strangers if it doesn't feel right?
- What would you say to the stranger?
- Do you think it's better for a child to help an adult, or for an adult to help an adult?
- What should you do if an adult asks you to help them and there is noone around to help?

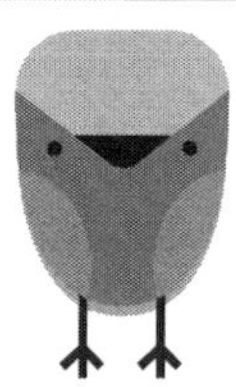

The Victim, the Bully and the Bystander

Where does the potential for bullying exist? Wherever there is a power imbalance. Over 50% of 8 year olds say that bullying is a big problem in schools. Often, this manifests as children teasing one another due to differences such as skin colour, culture or physical appearance. It's important your child understands that this is completely inappropriate behaviour.

Empathy

Teaching empathy and assertiveness is the best way to prevent your child from bullying others.

Ask questions like:

- *How would you feel if someone did that to you?*
- *How do you think that made the other person feel?*

Putting them in the other kid's shoes encourages thoughtfulness and empathy.

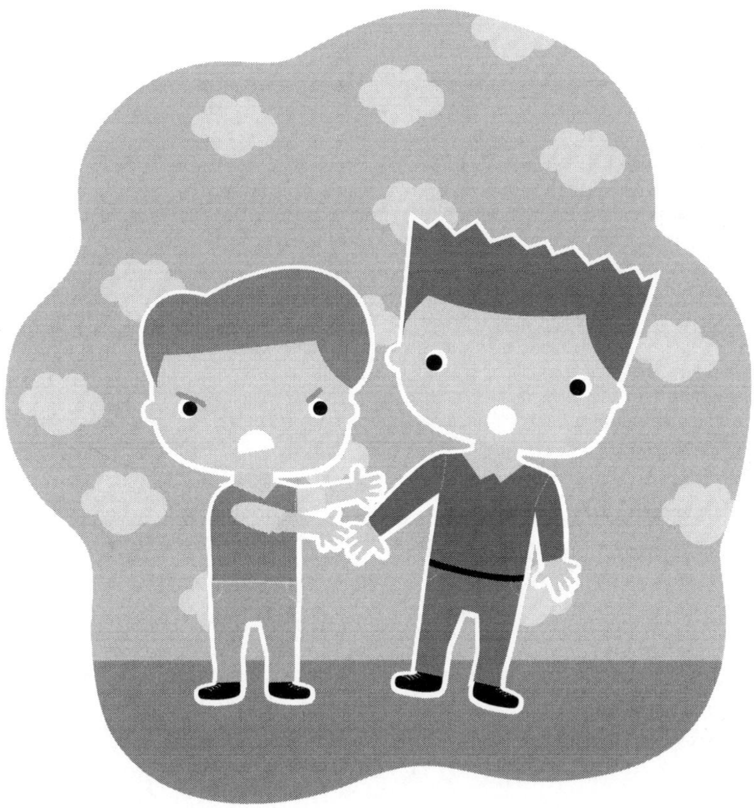

Say No!

Empower your child to say NO so that if they encounter bullying, they won't feel forced to do anything against their wishes. Teach basic "I" Statements that will assist them in expressing how others' behaviour makes them feel:

- *I don't like it when you make fun of me, it makes me feel...*

When your kid does something good, praise their behaviour! When they act inappropriately, discipline with consistency. Bullying can include another child asking to see their private parts. Depending if coercion is occurring, investigate further. Calmly ask what's prompting these actions. Curiosity? Something else? How the child answers will indicate whether the situation warrants a conversation with their parents.

Modelling

Children model their behaviour on the actions of the adults in their lives, picking up on every nuance, look, action, attitude and verbal cue. Consistently celebrate difference and diversity when interacting with your child! Don't ignore bullying, especially between siblings or children of disparate ages. Your kid needs to understand that bullying is not acceptable and will be disciplined accordingly. Tolerating bullying sends the message that you think it's okay. Keep your eyes open! Bickering or fighting is a natural part of development, but it can lead to more aggressive behaviour, often escalating into violence if ignored.

The Bystander

Teach them the power of the bystander / witness. Even if they're not in the firing line, many children are reluctant to intervene when they see someone being bullied because they're afraid of what will happen to them, they think they'll make the situation worse, or they simply don't know what to do!

If they cannot confront the bully directly, they should tell you, a teacher, or a trusted adult what transpired. Bullying in schools is woefully under-reported because children think it's wrong to do so. They're afraid to be labelled as a *squealer/tattle tail,* but the best way to help everyone involved (the bully included) is to engage, educate, empathize and empower all parties. They need to know that it's okay to tell when bullying is involved.

Encourage your children to believe in themselves, more importantly reinforce that you believe in them. Teach them the skills they need to protect themselves socially, then let them know that you trust them to make good judgements. Tell them that you love them and show them how important they are to you. Children who know that they're cared for, can think for themselves and have a strong sense of self worth rarely feel the need to bully someone else and are in turn not picked on by bullies.

Build empathy by getting them to imagine what it would feel like if they were in that person's shoes.

START THE CONVERSATION ...

- What is bullying?
- What does a bully do?
- How do you think people feel that are being bullied?
- Do you know any bullies?
- What do you do if someone is bullying you?
- Has anyone tried to bully you?
- Have you tried to bully someone? Why?
- Do you think bullying is a good thing to do?
- What would you say or do if you saw someone being bullied?
- When you don't let another child play with you or your group of friends is that bullying?
- When someone is mean to someone else because they're different, is that bullying?
- What makes people different? Special?

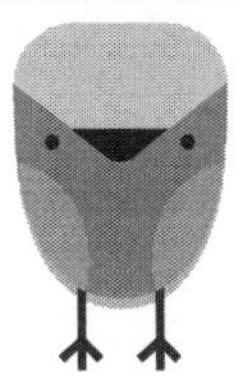

BOTTOM LINE:

- **Not only does your child need to understand the names and functions of their private parts. They need learn their rights and identify their boundaries as well.**
- **Explain that it's inappropriate for anyone to touch or kiss their private parts or for them to touch or kiss the private parts of others.**
- **Make sure they understand that if anyone tells them this behaviour is okay or to keep it a secret, that it's wrong.**
- **Sexual abuse is a sensitive topic. It's more common than most people think so being educated on what to look for is important.**
- **Self-stimulation and exploration is completely normal and healthy behaviour that should be done in private, not public.**
- **Exploration with other children is normal for this age but children should be reminded that their private parts are special and shouldn't be shared.**
- **Only a small percentage of children are harmed by strangers but it's important to arm your children with the tools to protect themselves and stay safe.**
- **Don't ignore bullying, your child needs to understand that bullying is not acceptable and will be disciplined accordingly. Tolerating bullying sends the message that you think it's okay.**

In the next section....
Children within this age group begin to understand that in addition to physical differences, there are other differences between genders and start to question how they fit in. However, not all children fit neatly into stereotypical gender roles.

Who Am I ? Where Do I Fit In?

During their formative years, kids learn about sex from the attitudes, mannerisms and non-verbal cues that their parents exhibit. But as they grow, children begin drawing conclusions from their ever-expanding world as well.

You may start to notice certain behaviours that are perfectly normal for this age group but upsetting to you, nonetheless! For instance, your child may develop strong feelings for other children of their gender, which is actually quite typical of this age – feelings which sometimes lead to same-sex exploration.

Sexual Diversity

Kids this age are aware of the physical differences between the sexes along with the gender biases society propagates for each. Although everyone is born male or female, not everyone identifies with their biological gender nor is attracted to the opposite sex.

As you can imagine, this can be a confusing time for kids, especially when they become exposed to the range of opinions about sexual orientation. Likely, they've already seen same-sex couples holding hands and heard labels such as *gay, lesbian,* or *queer.*

What makes it even more confusing is that strong feelings aren't always indicative of a physical or romantic connection.

Where to start?

There are three things every child should know:

- sexual orientation is not a choice
- ALL people deserve respect, regardless of their sexual orientation
- who someone is attracted to is only a small part of who they are

Once they've taken these fundamental truths to heart, encourage their questions!

Who's Who

Explain that people who feel physically / romantically attracted to members of the opposite sex are considered *heterosexual,* those who feel physically / romantically attracted to members of the same sex are considered *homosexual,* and those with feelings for both are considered *bisexual.*

The term *gay* is sometimes used to refer to homosexual men and the term *lesbian* to homosexual women.

Never comment negatively about the sexual orientations of others. Instilling judgments about any aspect of someone else's values and beliefs only teaches disrespect, intolerance and ignorance. If your child is struggling with how they feel about the same sex (confusion can happen this young) negative language will only alienate them giving them feelings of isolation.

Want your kid to have a healthy perspective? Teach facts, not opinions! Express to your child that you love them no matter who they are or become in the future.

START THE CONVERSATION ...

- Do you know what gay means? Bisexual?
- How do you think a gay person is different from others? How do you think they're the same as others?
- Have you heard anyone say anything about LGBTQ people? What do you think about what they said?
- Do you have any friends that have two moms or two dads?
- Does anyone say anything to you about having two moms/two dads?
- Do you have any questions about boys who like boys or girls who like girls?

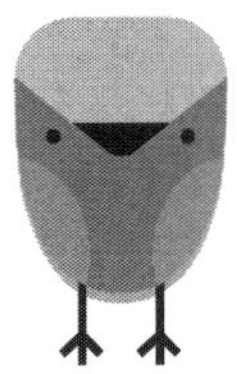

Gender Identity

By age eight, most kids have already developed a sense of gender identity (the awareness that they are female or male) and gender consistency (the awareness that they're going to stay that way). But for a small percentage of children, it's not so easy. Confusingly, a child's sex (identity based upon their genitals) can differ from their gender (identity based upon their perception of being a male or female).

If you child consistently expresses that they identify with the gender opposite of their genitalia, it may be that they're *transgendered* or a *gender-variant*. Be clear that being transgendered has nothing to do with sexual orientation. It simply means that the child feels different from the biologic sex their genitals reflect. Gender-variants are people who do not conform to any gender and have behaviours and interests that don't typically align with a specific gender. They may enjoy being a girl one day and a boy the next. Some children don't have a connection to either gender, which can be even more confusing.

It's not a choice to be transgendered or a gender-variant! People are born that way. Being a transgendered or a gender-variant boy can be particularly hard since societal norms tend to be

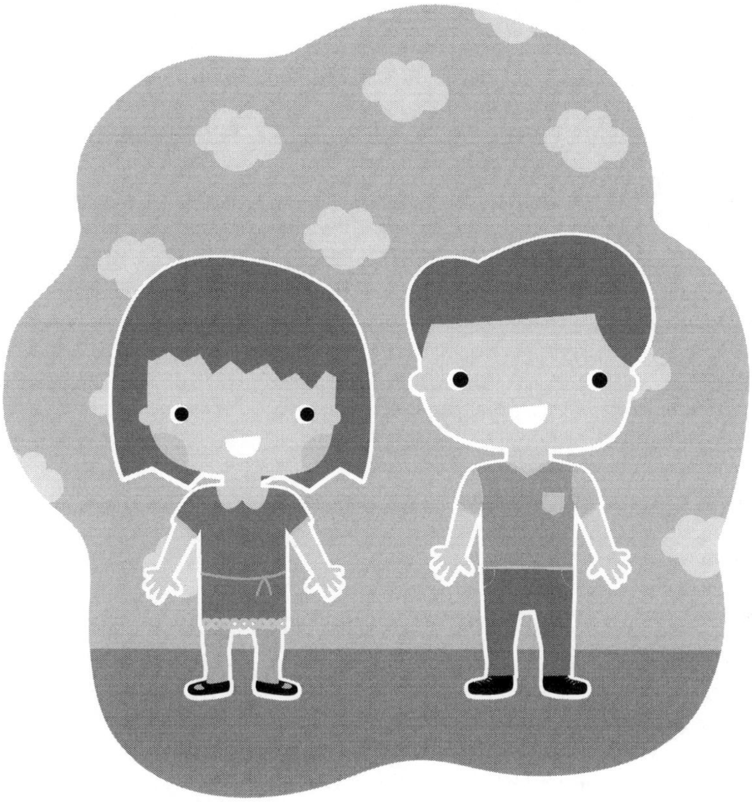

less flexible for males. A girl with a short haircut and boys clothes blends in much better than a boy with long hair and a dress. Acknowledge your child's strengths and encourage, support, and celebrate them as an individual, not as a boy or a girl.

Raising a Transgender/Gender-Variant Child

Suspecting that your child is transgendered can be very upsetting as a parent, which is why you need to remind yourself that your kid's going through much more than you are! Reassure them that you love them unconditionally and want them to be exactly who they are. They'll need your support more than ever to navigate what lies ahead.

Don't try to change their behaviour! No one chooses to be a gender-variant or transgendered person. Pressure to conform can lead to embarrassment, shame, behavioural issues, violence, and even thoughts of suicide.

Don't be ashamed if you're having a hard time dealing and don't be afraid to reach out! Often, the whole family needs support during this challenging transition. The road to acceptance is long and often painful for all involved but for the sake of your kid, it can't be ignored.

START THE CONVERSATION ...

- We love you the way you are and always will. You're special because there is no one else like you in the whole world and we are proud of you.

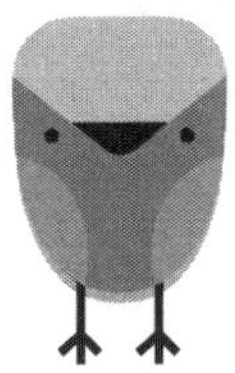

Stereotypes

Usually, children in this age group have already developed pronounced perceptions of stereotypical gender roles. Culture, media, religion, and personal experiences influence all of our perceptions and categorization is a natural means of rationalizing our world – but that doesn't necessarily make it healthy nor accurate!

Because we make assumptions based on our own frame of reference (i.e. what we were taught to perceive as normal) we automatically attempt to protect our children from being ostracized by encouraging them to adopt this idea of normal, too.

Chances are, you're unaware of the stereotypes you encourage. It's important to remember that (regardless of what belief system you subscribe to) children shouldn't be forced into doing anything that makes them feel uncomfortable. Some of your child's behaviours might be environment-influenced (nurture) but many are inherent (nature) too. Respect what can't be changed!

Your approach to gender stereotyping will have lasting affects on the way your child feels about themselves and others. Some stereotypes they'll encounter include:

Girls

- *wear pink*
- *wear dresses*
- *have long hair*
- *play with dolls*
- *skip rope*
- *express verbally*
- *can cry*

Boys

- *wear blue*
- *wear pants*
- *have short hair*
- *play with balls*
- *enjoy team sports*
- *express physically*
- *don't cry*

Let your kid explore their individuality by expressing it in a way that for them comes naturally. Pay attention to their strengths, celebrating them as an individual rather than as a boy or a girl. Seize every teachable moment as an opportunity to discuss the differences between boys and girls, explaining that (physicality aside) neither sex has to conform to these stereotypes. Most importantly, reassure them that it's fine to be different and that everyone is born unique and special in their own way.

Strategies

Encourage your child to treat others as individuals, correcting them if they make gender-specific statements and suggesting situation-specific or person-specific ways of expressing their feelings. No one should judge anyone else because of the way they look, the color of their skin, the clothes they wear or the sport they play. Model good behaviour! Your kid looks to you for guidance and will copy what you say and do, which is why it's so important to back up your words with your actions. If you tell your child that it's normal for both parents to do the ironing, make sure that both parents do!

Remind your child that if they're teased for their appearance or their actions it's considered bullying and should be reported to a parent or teacher immediately!

Don't pressure them to be something they're not. You're not protecting your child by forcing them to fit into a certain stereotype, you're doing them a disservice. Remember that sexuality is a dynamic process that continues to develop and change throughout life. Your job as a parent is to encourage them to be who they want to be and celebrate who they are.

If your daughter isn't comfortable wearing dresses but opts for pants and a tee shirt instead, support her unique personality rather than pressuring her to *dress like a girl.* If you find your son wearing his sister's dress, it probably doesn't indicate sexual confusion. Sometimes, it's just a manifestation of innocent curiosity. Children enjoy experimenting with different roles and need the room and support to do so.

START THE CONVERSATION ...

- Do you think boys can wear pink? Can girls can play with trucks?
- What do you think is special about being a boy or girl? Tell your child how they are special in their own way.
- Is there anything that girls/boys do that you feel you can't do because you're not a boy/girl?
- What games do the boys and girls play at school?
- You don't like wearing dresses. How would you like to dress?

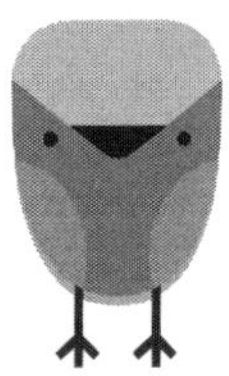

BOTTOM LINE:

- **Don't make negative remarks about the sexual orientations of others in front of your children. Judgments about any aspect of someone else's values and beliefs only teaches disrespect, intolerance and ignorance.**
- **Forcing a child to be something they're not or failing to acknowledge them for who they are can have a negative effect on their sense of self worth.**
- **Transgendered or gender variant children are born that way.**
- **Transgendered children do not identify with the sex they were born into.**
- **Gender variant children do not identify with either male or female gender.**
- **Don't force your child to conform to stereotypes.**
- **Celebrate your child as an individual and encourage them to do the same.**

In the next section....
Parents and siblings are the key influencers in children's lives as they learn their family's dynamic and discover their role in it. Whether experiencing curiosity about their bodies, negotiating new friendships or grappling with divorce, it's important that you're aware of their thoughts and feelings.

Making Connections

Family Diversity

Families come in many different shapes, sizes and forms. Some have a male and female parent while others have one parent, two same-sex parents, or even other family members acting as parents. Explain to your child that every family is unique, made up of people who love one another regardless of the circumstances that created them. Celebrate these differences with your child! Children are unique too. Some are biologically connected to their families while others are adopted or fostered. It's important to remember that all families are equal because they are composed of people who love and care for one another regardless of sexual orientation, age, race, gender, culture, or religion.

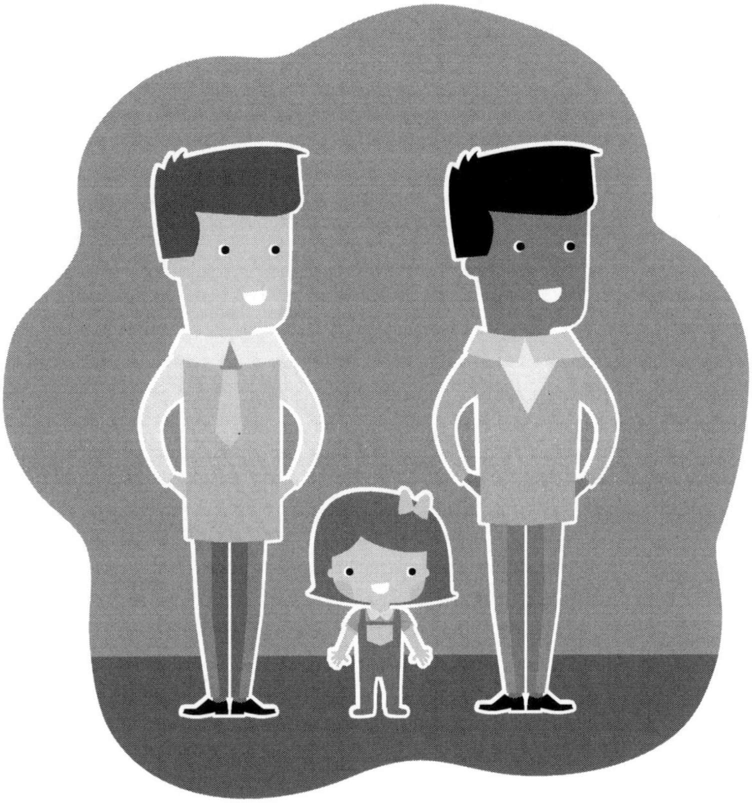

Dealing With Divorce and Separation

Divorce and separation are very traumatic for kids because they learn far more from your actions and attitudes than you realize.

Seeing parents in emotional conflict can be devastating for a child and have far-reaching effects on how they view relationships throughout their lives. Parents who are going through a divorce are often so involved in their own misery that they can overlook the fact that their
... may feel that they did or didn't do something to cause the split. You see, children aren't
...derstand why their parents no longer want to be together and often fear that
...ned by one parent or that one loves them less than the other.
...id that both parents still love them and will always be part of their lives (pro-

vided that's the case). Regardless of the circumstances, they need to understand that what's occurring isn't their fault. Try to have this dialogue as a united parental front, no matter how painful it may be. Remember, this isn't about you! It's about them.

Keep the conversation simple and stick to the facts, letting them know what to expect and answering questions in a way that's age appropriate while still being respectful to your privacy too. If you let your child express their feelings, it will help them make sense of the situation and help you dispel the misconceptions that are certain to arise.

Never blame or malign your ex-partner in front of your child! All your child wants is to take your pain away. If you ignore the high road, they'll only take on your negativity, which will affect everyone's relationships moving forward. Remember that your child is your child, not your confidant. Don't rely on them for emotional support, counsel or as a shoulder to cry on.

Stepfamilies

Children find it hard to adapt to a new family dynamic when one or both parents remarry, especially if the transition involves step-siblings.

Do you have a new partner? Be patient if your child doesn't fall in love with them (and theirs) immediately. As far as your kid's concerned, this person's a stranger, which means they'll need time to develop trust and familiarity. Respect that!

Children often experience anger toward one or both parents for the divorce or separation and it may be hard for them to see you move on, particularly if they secretly harbor hopes of a happy reunion, a-la The Parent Trap. There's nothing Disney about a divorce and it's your job to break that reality gently.

START THE CONVERSATION ...

- How do you feel about the change that is happening in our family? Reassure..
- Please share your feelings with me. It's okay.

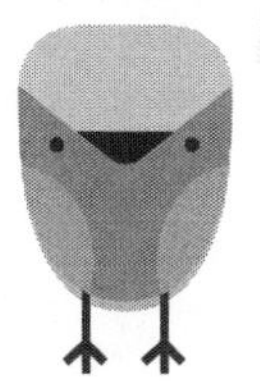

Brothers and Sisters

Children turn to those closest to them for guidance, and the relationships they forge with siblings often sets the stage for their behaviour in other relationships. Older siblings can be great sharers of wisdom and younger ones can be excellent objects of empathy. Of course, sibling squabbling is normal too and every altercation is an excellent opportunity to learn something. Just be sure to monitor behaviour and preempt power imbalances that could turn to bullying.

Strategies

There's a difference between bullying and bickering! Bullying involves power imbalance, repetition, and a negative emotional response from the victim. You'll need to remain vigilant in order to differentiate between the two. Stop bullying between siblings the minute you notice it and reinforce empathy and boundaries.

Treat all your children equally and never pick favourites or play one against the other. Encourage honest communication and mutual respect by reinforcing good behaviour with enthusiastic praise. Don't ignore bullying! If you don't nip bad behaviour in the bud, you're sending the message that it's acceptable, which will only lead to progressively more aggressive behaviour.

Best Friends Forever

As children in this age group begin developing relationships with people outside of their family, they begin discovering the vast assortment of dynamics that exist and find independence venturing into new physical and emotional territory of their own. The problem is it makes them very vulnerable as they discover guidelines for appropriate behaviour and establish boundaries on their own terms. This is when your kid will form intimate same-sex relationships and probably find that first best friend who'll teach them how to navigate feelings and emotions in this context.

Strategies

Relationship building is a learned skill! Support the forging of new friendships through participation in social activities like birthday parties and play-dates.

Remind your child that friendships are based on mutual respect, honesty and trust. Support their uniqueness and remind them that diversity in their friend group is something to celebrate!

This process is much harder for some kids than others. Monitor your child's interactions closely, stressing the importance of sharing, caring, and empathy while reinforcing that real friends don't coerce, tease, or bully each other. Remind them to tell you (or another trusted adult) immediately if they become victim to this type of behaviour.

Don't force your child into uncomfortable social situations. Anxious children take longer to warm up to other children and may benefit more from one-on-one play-dates in quiet places. Immerse yourself in your child's world! Get to know their school environment, their friends' families, your neighbours, and any newcomers into their lives. If you're aware of what and whom your child is exposed to, you'll be able to ensure that the situations and interactions they experience are consistent with the values and beliefs you wish to instil.
Encourage *supervised independence*. By exercising due diligence with situations involving new people and scenarios, you'll give your child the opportunity to grow without continually hovering over them.

When Dreams Become Nightmares

Dreaming is our brain's way of subconsciously processing emotions and experiences but sometimes the subject matter can turn them into nightmares. Nightmares aren't always attributed to specific reasons but in children, they can be brought on by factors as simple as change or stress. Don't go light on the compassion when a nightmare wakes your child! Offering comfort shows that you understand their fear and that it's okay for them to feel this emotion. Reassure them that you're there and that what they experienced didn't happen in

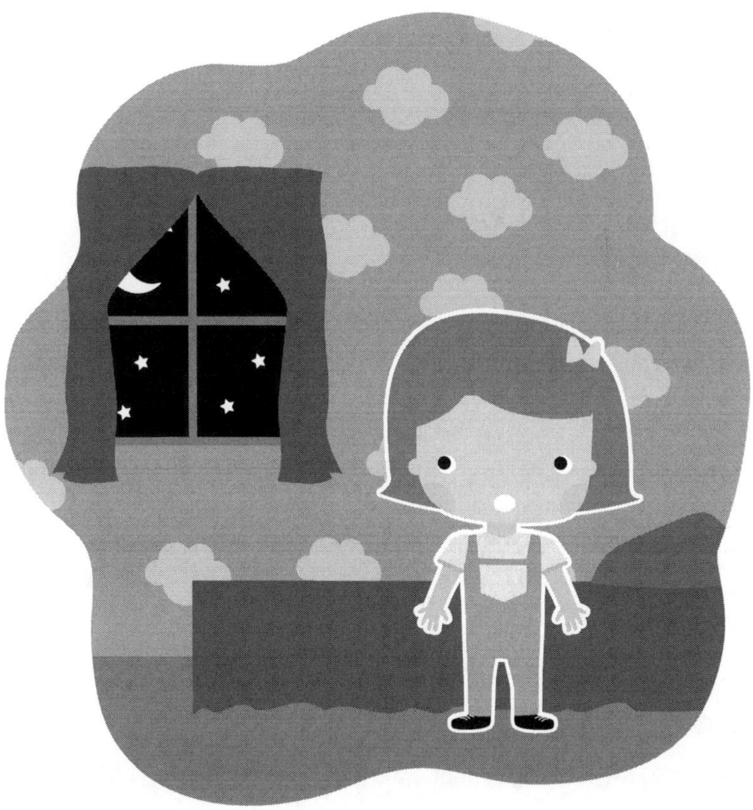

the real world. If a nightlight or hall light makes them feel better, leave one on. Once they've calmed down and feel safe, they'll be ready to go back to sleep.
Generally, nightmares shouldn't be cause for concern but if they're happening persistently enough to affect your kid's sleep patterns or if they're associated with behavioural or emotional concerns, play it safe and see a doctor.

Please Don't Leave Me!

Separation Anxiety is distress brought on by separation from a parent/primary caregiver. Usually, separation anxiety disappears with time but it can occasionally continue into the elementary school years.
If your child suddenly displays symptoms of separation anxiety after years without, the distress may be rooted elsewhere. Be aware of situations that may indicate bullying or abuse. If your kid consistently refuses to go to school or to be babysat by the same person, it could be an indication of a greater underlying problem. Happy, content kids shouldn't feel unsafe when their parents aren't present.
Separation Anxiety Disorder is a very real thing, too.

If your child's anxiety persists beyond the elementary school years, they might be struggling with something that a doctor is best equipped to deal with.

I'm So Fat!

Due to media's daily barrage of sex and sexualized messaging, kids quickly begin making connections between appearance and value. As they learn society's physical criteria for beauty, they begin comparing their bodies to those around them. This is a dangerous game that for many kids, results in body image issues.
Bodies (like families) come in many different shapes and sizes and there's no such thing as an ideal body type any more than there is such thing as an ideal family type. In fact, a person's health and strength is far more important than what size of jeans they wear. Remind your kid that what they see and hear in the media is rarely representative of reality and not worth creating a comparison to. Showing them images of average, healthy bodies will go a long way in driving this message home!
Always lead by example! Regardless of your own body type (and hang-ups) complement yourself in the presence of your child with affirmations such as, *I feel and look great today!* What

you're doing is communicating confidence that isn't dependent upon image. In this context, it's easy to see why comments like, *I need to go on a diet, I'm so fat,* or *I look awful today,* can be so damaging.

Never feed your child's anxiety by confirming their body image misconceptions. If your child's unhealthily overweight/underweight, don't implement a change in their diet without first consulting a nutritionist!

Most importantly, remind your child at every opportunity that they are valued for their talents, abilities, and accomplishments – not because of how they look.

START THE CONVERSATION ...

- What makes up a family?
- What do you love about your family?
- How do you feel about a family having only a dad or mom, grandparents etc? Talk about their feelings, explore.
- People come in all shapes, sizes and colors. Tell me about all the friends in your life and how they are different?
- How are they the same?
- Do you think their insides are the same as yours?
- What are three things you love about yourself?
- Let me tell you about the things I love about you...
- Do you think that movie stars look like that all the time? Talk about airbrushing/makeup etc.
- What is special about you?
- Let me tell you what I love about myself. I think this makes me special...(model behaviour).
- How do you feel about mommy/daddy not being together any more? Why? Reinforce that you love them and that you understand what they're feeling.
- What do you think about mommy/daddy getting married to/living with someone else? Reinforce that they are special and will always be a part of your family.

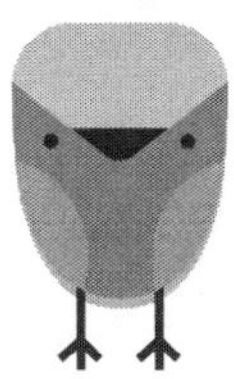

BOTTOM LINE:

- **Every family is unique, made up of people who love one another regardless of the circumstances that created them.**
- **Divorce isn't about you. It's about your children.**
- **Unlike sibling squabbling, bullying involves power imbalance, repetition, and a negative emotional response on the part of the victim.**
- **Support your child as they forge new friendships through participation in social activities.**
- **If your child suddenly displays symptoms of separation anxiety after years without, investigate.**
- **Nightmares can't always be attributed to a specific reason but can be catalyzed by factors as simple as change or stress.**
- **There's no such thing as an ideal body type, what children see and hear in the media isn't always real. Remind your children that they should be valued for who they are as an individual, not based on their physical appearance.**
- **Don't put yourself down in front of your kids, model the behaviour and attitude you want them to display with a positive body image.**

In the next section....

What you've all been waiting for.... What to tell your Primary school children about the Birds and the Bees...

THE TRUTH ABOUT MAKING BABIES

If your child hasn't asked you about reproduction and pregnancy yet, it's time for you to initiate the conversation yourself. This dialogue often doubles as damage control, since most kids have acquired at least one misconception by this age about sex, pregnancy and childbirth from their peers!

It's likely that they've seen countless pregnant women, prompting the thoughts (if not the questions) *How are babies born? Where did I come from? Did you do that?*

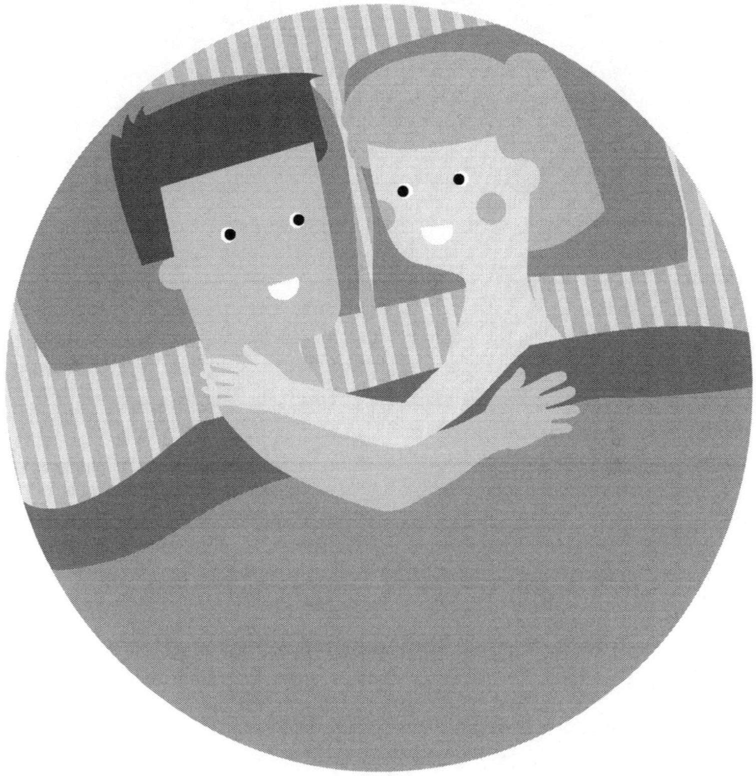

Many parents are concerned that sexually educating their child at a young age leads to early sexual activity or promiscuity later in life. However, studies show that children who are taught about sex early tend to delay sexual activity. It's ignorance coupled with curiosity (not knowledge) that leads to earlier sexual experimentation.

Be Honest!

Babies don't come from the hospital or the stork! Telling your child that they do will only undermine your credibility as a reliable source of information when your child discovers the truth elsewhere (and they will). Don't excuse your child from school lessons on sexual health either. If you're feeling uncomfortable, talk with their educator so you're aware what will be taught and can follow up with your child accordingly.

It's more effective to have many little talks along the way than one big *Talk*, which usually happens too late for most children. Explain the basics of reproduction, going into as much detail as you are comfortable with and watching for cues from your child that indicate when their curiosity has been satisfied.

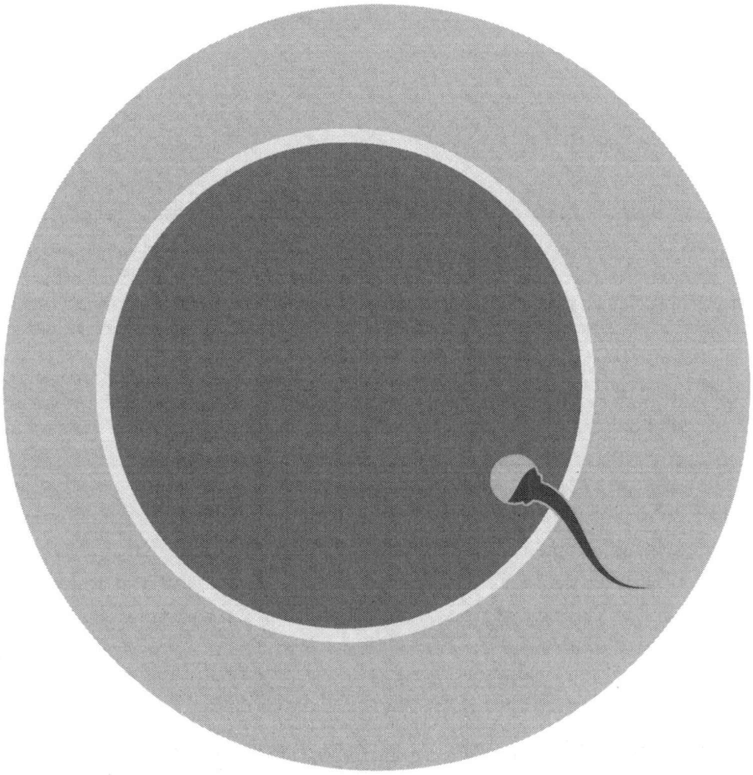

Teach your child that babies can only be made when a seed (sperm) from a man joins with an egg (ovum) from a woman when they hold each other in a special way which is called having sex. Most commonly, babies are made during sex (the act of putting the penis into the vagina) when a man's sperm joins with a woman's egg. Babies, can also be made using IVF or *in vitro* fertillization by joining a sperm from a man with an egg from a woman outside of their bodies. Once the sperm and egg have joined, they're put back into the mother's womb.

As the baby grows in the womb it is surrounded by water (amniotic fluid) which protects the baby. A special cord called the *umbilical cord* attaches from the mommy to the baby. This is how the mommy gives the baby the food it needs to grow and helps it "breathe".

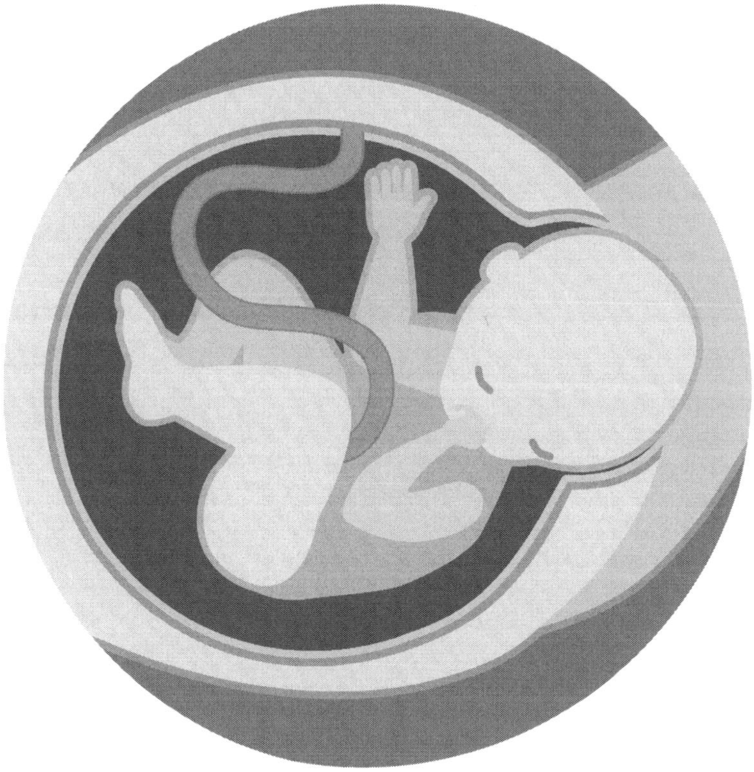

The baby continues to grow inside the mother's womb which makes it stretch outwards in front of her. The mother can start to feel when the baby moves around and sometimes it kicks!

When the baby is ready to be born, the mother's womb starts to push down around the baby (contract)

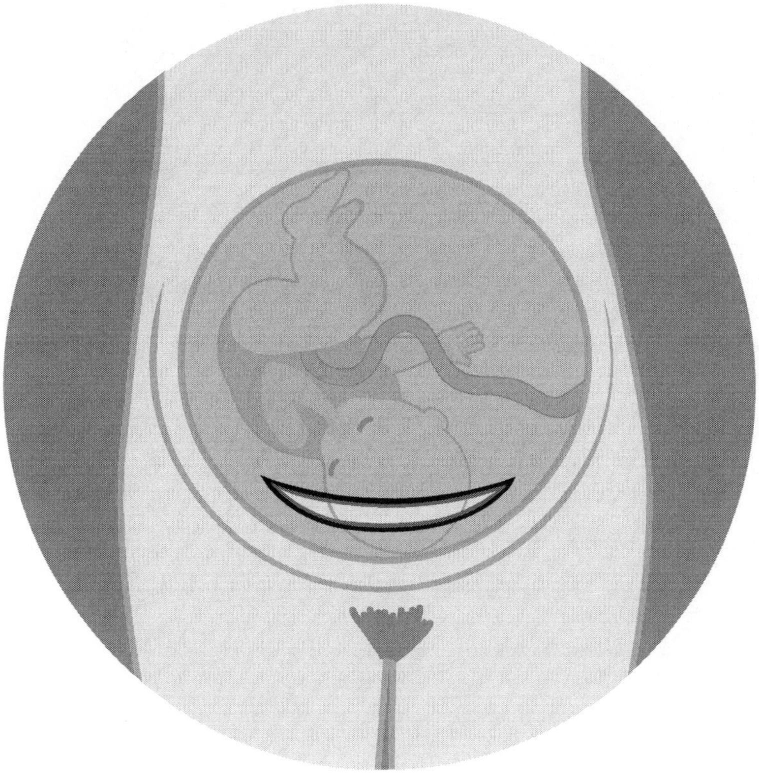

like a great big hug to help it to move through the vagina (which stretches like an elastic to let the baby through and then goes back to it's normal size) and come out of the mother's body on a water slide.

Sometimes the hug isn't strong enough so the doctor makes a cut in the mother's tummy (called a Cesarean or C-Section) and takes the baby out from there. The doctor gives the mother medicine so the cut doesn't hurt.

Once the baby is out of the mother's body and can breath on it's own, the doctor cuts the umbilical cord. This doesn't hurt the mother or the baby and a few days later the little bit of cord that was left on the baby falls off on it own, leaving a bellybutton or navel behind!

Sometimes more than one baby grows inside the mother's womb. When two babies are conceived (made) and born at the same time, they're called twins.

Twins are made in two ways (See illustrations on following page) *:*

- **Fraternal Twins** ~ *when two eggs get fertilized by two sperm at the same time. These twins don't look exactly alike and can be a boy and a girl.*

- **Identical Twins** ~ *when an egg gets fertilized by one sperm but soon after the baby starts to develop it splits into two. These twins look exactly alike and can only be two boys or two girls.*

Quick Answers for Kids has the answers to the many more questions your kids might ask about sex, reproduction and childbirth.

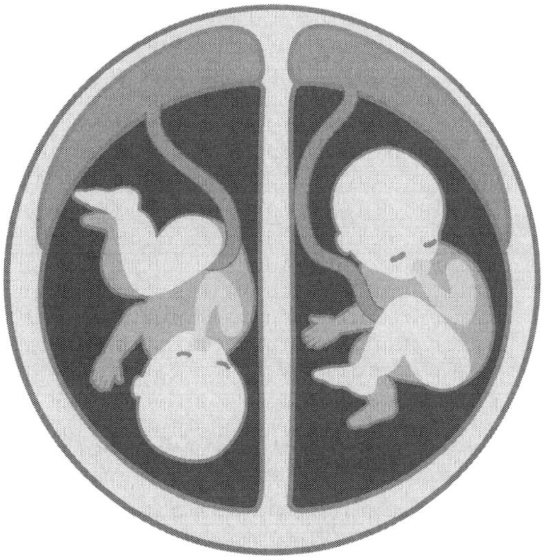

Fraternal Twins

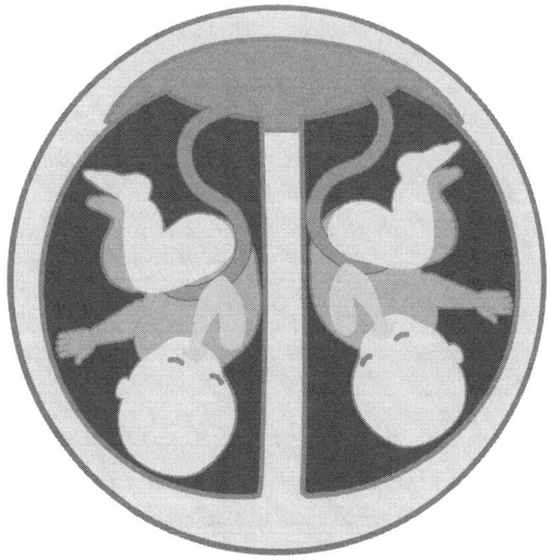

Identical Twins

START THE CONVERSATION ...

- Why do you ask?
- What do you think?
- What have you heard?
- What do you think a sperm is?
- What do you think an ovum/egg is?
- How do you think the sperm reaches the egg?
- Where do you think the penis has to go to reach the egg?
- Can you name the place where the baby grows?
- What questions do you have?
- Where does the baby grow?
- Can you guess how long it takes to grow?
- Can you guess what that cord is for?
- How do you think the baby can eat or breath?
- Do you know what twins are? There are two different types of twins. How are they different?
- Do you know any twins?
- Do they look alike or do they look different?
- Babies are born two different ways. Do you know how?
- Can you name two ways the baby can leave the womb?

A Word on Condoms and HIV

Condoms

Unfortunately, it's all too common to find used condoms in places like playgrounds and parks. It's important that children understand what they are and why they can't touch them.
Both men and women can wear condoms (men on their penises and women in their vaginas) but in both cases their functionality's the same:

- *to block a man's sperm from coming in contact with a woman's egg*
- *to stop the spread of germs from one person to another*

Condoms are clean and healthy when adults buy them from the store but have germs on them after they've been used. Because germs make people sick, children mustn't pick up condoms. If they find one, it's important that they know to report it to a trusted adult immediately.

HIV

Whether through the media, peers or older siblings, it's likely that your kid's heard a few things about HIV. Often, this limited grasp of the subject leads to misconceptions and irrational fears. Some of them may have classmates with HIV and worry that it's contagious. They might think they can get it by touching people who have it or using the same public bathroom. Which is why it's important that they know a little bit about it.
HIV (Human Immunodeficiency Virus) is a viral infection that lives in bodily fluids (i.e. blood, semen, vaginal fluid, breast milk, eye fluid) and is spread by the exchange of these fluids with someone who's already infected. This usually happens during sex but sometimes during the accidental exchange of blood (i.e. un-sanitized tattoo needles and needle sharing among intravenous drug-users).
Reassure your child that they're not at risk of contracting HIV since they're not engaging in

sexual activity, nor getting tattoos or using intravenous drugs. The needles that doctors and nurses use to administer medicine are always sanitized and never used more than once.

They may have heard of kids being born with HIV, which understandably, can lead to fears of infection. Be sure to let them know that in order for a baby to be born infected, the parents must be infected too.

There's really no need to scare or confuse your child with complicated explanations. In this age group, a general idea of HIV is explanation enough. Never associate HIV with homosexual activity! This virus is not exclusive to the gay community and perceptions have changed since its emergence in the 1980s. In fact, heterosexual women are the fastest growing infected demographic. The BOTTOM LINE? HIV can be transmitted to anyone who is participating in unprotected sex or using intravenous drugs.

START THE CONVERSATION ...

- Have you seen this in a park or playground before? Show picture of a condom
- What should you do if you see it?
- Why do you think it's important not to touch it? (Bad germs or bugs)
- What do you think it's used for?
- Is it clean in it's package?

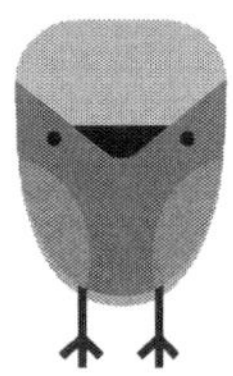

It's Only a Period!

Not surprisingly, kids have a lot of questions about menstruation. They're inundated with feminine hygiene commercials on the television, encounter products around the house and may even be in the bathroom when their mum's having a period.

Girls can experience their first period when they are as young as eight (although the average age is closer to 12 or 13) which is why it's important that your daughter understands menstruation and what to expect during this natural, healthy process *before* it happens.

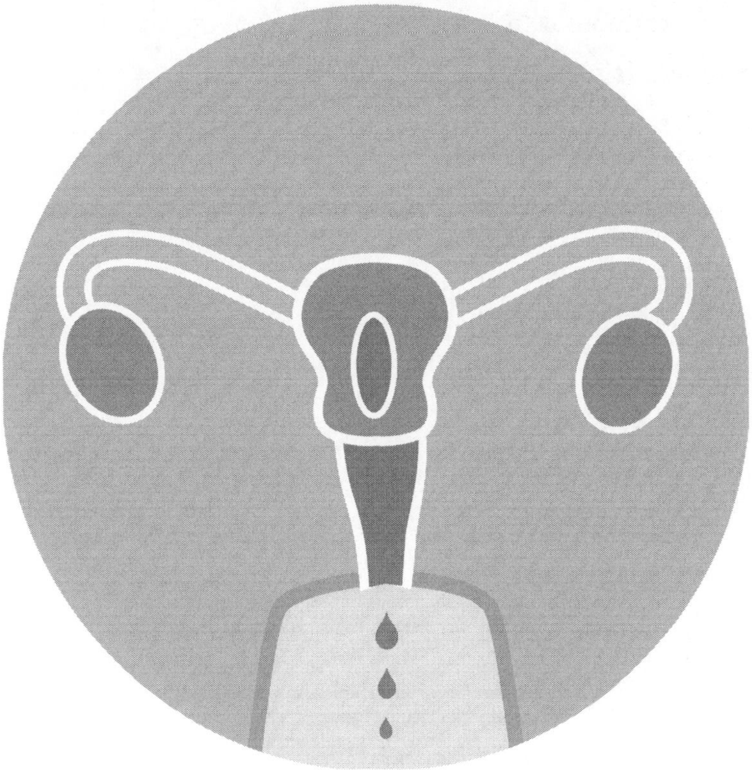

Explain to your daughter that menstruation is the body's way of preparing for reproduction. Once a month, the uterus grows a lining and when the female doesn't get pregnant, it leaves the uterus via the vagina in the form of drips.

These drips look like blood but they're actually mostly water and tiny bits of skin. Generally, periods occur monthly and the drips last for about a week at a time. Although this can some-

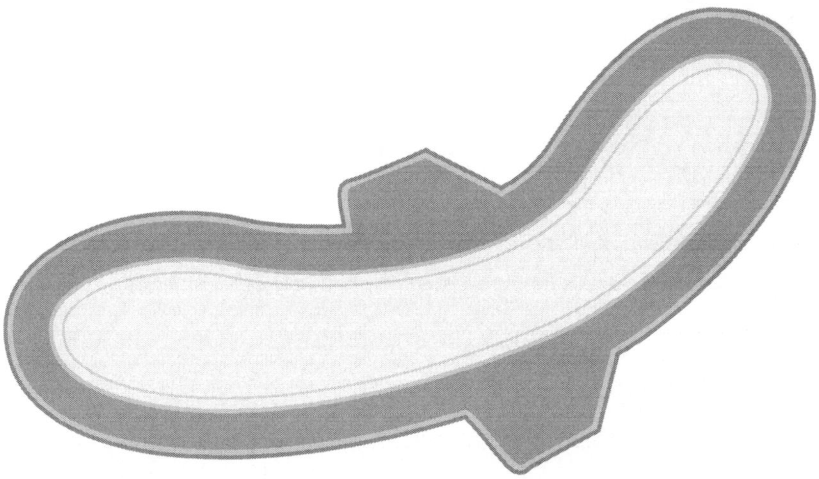

times cause pain in the abdominal area (cramps), there are lots of ways to control the discomfort.

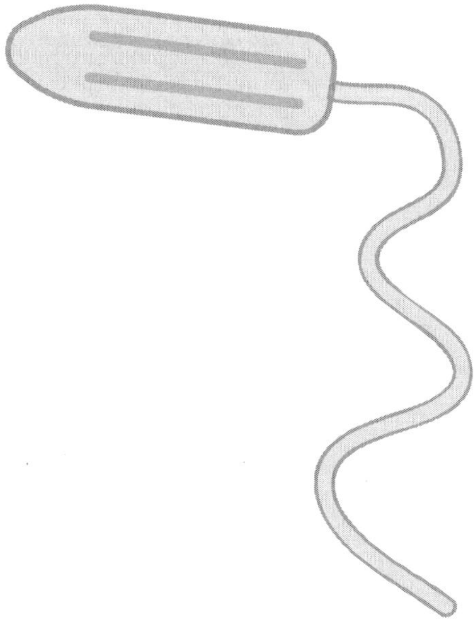

Your daughter should also understand the difference between pads, tampons and menstrual cups.

Pads (which come in the washable or disposable variety) are worn in the underwear to catch period drips from the outside of the body while tampons and menstrual cups are worn inside the vagina and serve the same purpose.

START THE CONVERSATION ...

- Where do you think the blood comes from? It's not all blood, let me explain..
- Why do you think girls have their period's?
- What do you think happens in the body?
- Do you think it happens to both boys and girls?
- When do you think it happens? (puberty)
- How do you feel about it?
- Does it scare you? Explain that it doesn't hurt
- Do you think it's normal? Explain that it's normal and all girls go through it.
- What do you think catches the drips when they come out of the body?
- Where do you think a tampon goes (show picture) to catch the drips?
- How do you think a pad (show picture) can be used to catch drips?
- Having your period is a very special event in a girl's life. Every girl starts her period. Some as young as 8 and others as old as 16. What do you know about getting your period?
- I'm so excited you asked me about your period! What a great question...

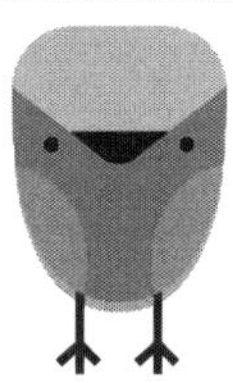

BOTTOM LINE:

- **Studies show that children who are taught about sex early by a trusted adult tend to delay sexual activity later in life.**
- **When talking to your child about reproduction, be honest and stick to the facts. Eventually they're going to learn the truth and being less than honest undermines their trust in you.**
- **Children need to know what condoms look like and not to pick up them up, because they could contain harmful germs.**
- **Reassure your child that they're not at risk of contracting HIV, because it can only be spread through sexual activity, or contact with contaminated needles.**
- **Menstruation is the way a girl's body gets ready for having a baby some day.**
- **It's a normal, natural and healthy thing and usually doesn't hurt, even though the drips might look like blood.**

In the next section....
Knowing about reproduction is only half the battle. Within this age group, children's exposure to various media increases exponentially and they need your help to put these messages into perspective based on your own family values.

Demystifying Media

Even in children aged 6-8, it's important for you to be conscious of what your child is hearing and seeing. After all, they're being inundated daily with information from movies, music, magazines, and television. Help them make sense of what they're experiencing!

TV

Don't underestimate television's dangerous potential as a miseducator. Not only does it reinforce limiting gender roles, it also imparts completely inaccurate facts (and all in the name of entertainment). Not all teenagers have sex, not everyone makes a lot of noise during sex and sex isn't violent! TV doesn't always represent reality. Even reality TV!

Limit the amount of TV watched as a family and whenever possible, strive to supervise your child's TV viewing and Internet use. Setting content and duration boundaries now will go a long way to negate future arguments. Teach your kid to be a critical viewer by engaging them about what they're watching. TV shows, movies, news, and even advertisements provide countless opportunities for teaching moments that illustrate the differences between reality, entertainment, and marketing.

Even full-time parents can't be parents full-time! For those times when duties take you elsewhere, block the channels / websites that contain explicit content, instate a permission first policy with PG-rated movies, and keep all devices in public areas of the home.

Social Media

Children are beginning to use social media at a younger and younger age. Most commonly, this begins with game consul networks and tube-uploaded TV shows. Due to its accessibility, this type of media often exposes children (of even the most vigilant parents) to age-inappropriate content.

Monitor your kid's usage of social media and don't allow them to maintain any accounts for which you don't have access. Ensure that you're aware of what they're watching online and with whom they're gaming. Set passwords on their behalf and reserve the right to check their activity when you see fit! Most importantly, let your child know that you trust them to make good decisions when you're not present and take an active, verbal role if they inadvertently view age-inappropriate content.

Internet

Thanks to the popularity of interactive games and online teaching tools, children as young as three are beginning to use the Internet. But it's all too easy for an innocent search query to come back with completely age-inappropriate page results. The solution? Online filtering software. Numerous products exist, all affordably priced and available to download. Remember, these programs aren't perfect. Nothing can take the place of in-person monitoring!

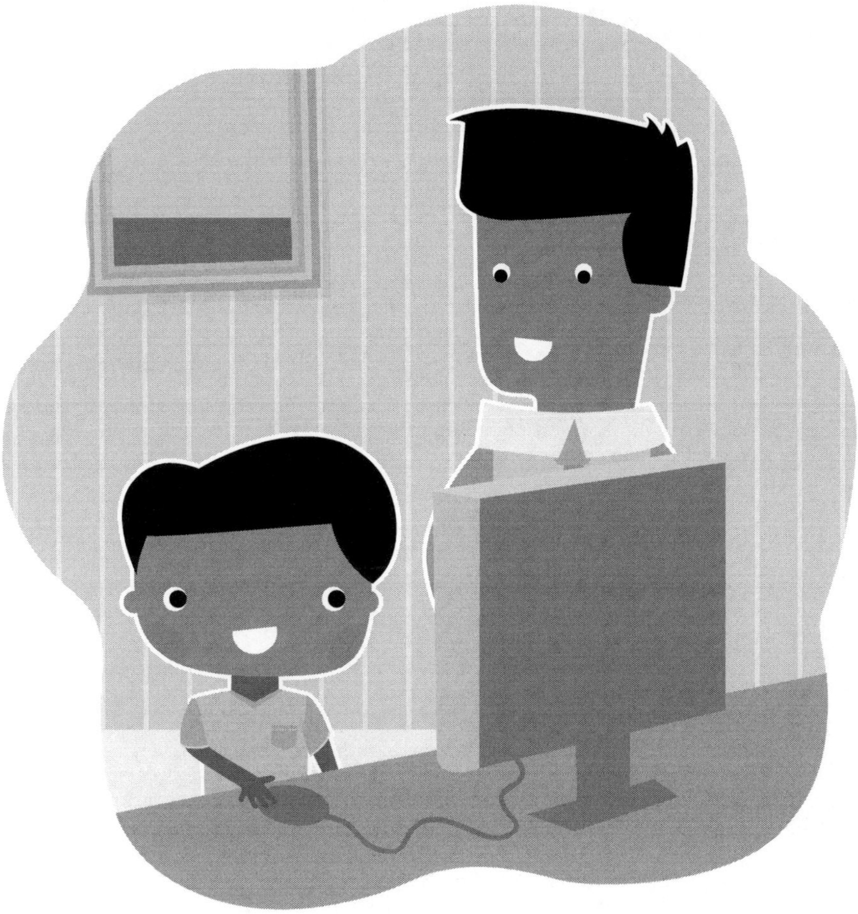

Music

Music tracks/videos are rife with explicit lyrics, violence, and sexual content. Stay up-to-date with your child's viewing and listening habits! If a song is derogatory, explicit, or misleading, regulate your child's exposure and explain how the content is inappropriate. Don't allow your child to download songs/videos if the content is contradictory to your values and beliefs.

START THE CONVERSATION ...

- Do you think things on TV are real?
- What do you think about the boys and girls you see on TV?
- What's your favorite show? Why?
- Do you have any questions about any shows you've watched?
- Do you know what an actor/actress is?
- What are your friend's favorite shows?
- Are there any shows you think I wouldn't like you watching? Why?
- What should you do if something you don't understand comes on the screen?
- Do you know what social media is? Let me explain....
- Do you think it's safe to talk to people over the internet? Discuss safety
- What if someone contacts you over the internet?
- Do you think it's easier to say something to someone online than it is in person?
- When do you think using the internet is appropriate?
- We should have some rules around the internet. What do you think they should be?
- Why should we have rules for using the internet?
- Do you think it's safe to share pictures of you over the internet?
- Where do you think they go?
- Do you think you can get them back?
- What kind of music do you like?
- Can you sing me part of the song?
- Why do you like the song?
- Do you know what your friends like?
- Who is your favorite singer? Why?
- Do you know what the words mean?
- What do you think they're like in real life?
- Do you think some words can mean more than one thing? Can you think of one in a song?
- What do you think of songs with bad words in them?
- Have you heard any? Tell me about it.

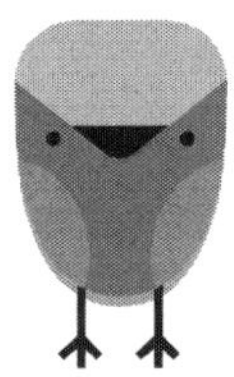

BOTTOM LINE:

- **Children are continually bombarded with sexual messages through the media and it's up to you as their parent to translate those messages to reflect your families values and beliefs.**
- **Teach your kid to be a critical viewer by engaging them about what they're seeing and hearing.**
- **Keep up to date on changing technology. Parents need to understand the full capabilities and power of the gadgets their children are using.**

In the next section...
For those of you who may be wondering what sorts of questions children in this age group have, or what questions other parents are asking... Our experts have put together some of the toughest questions kids and parents ask… and provided the answers!

60 Quick Answers to Tough Questions

51 Quick Answers for Kids:

1. **Can two boys get married?**
   Yes. In Canada, it's legal for two men or two women in a gay relationship to get married. In the United States the laws vary within each state.

2. **Why does my friend have two mums?**
   Your friend's mums are gay but they are parents exactly like a mum and a dad are. One of the things that make families so wonderful is how different each and every one is.

3. **What are twins?**
   Twins are two babies that are conceived(made) and born at the same time.

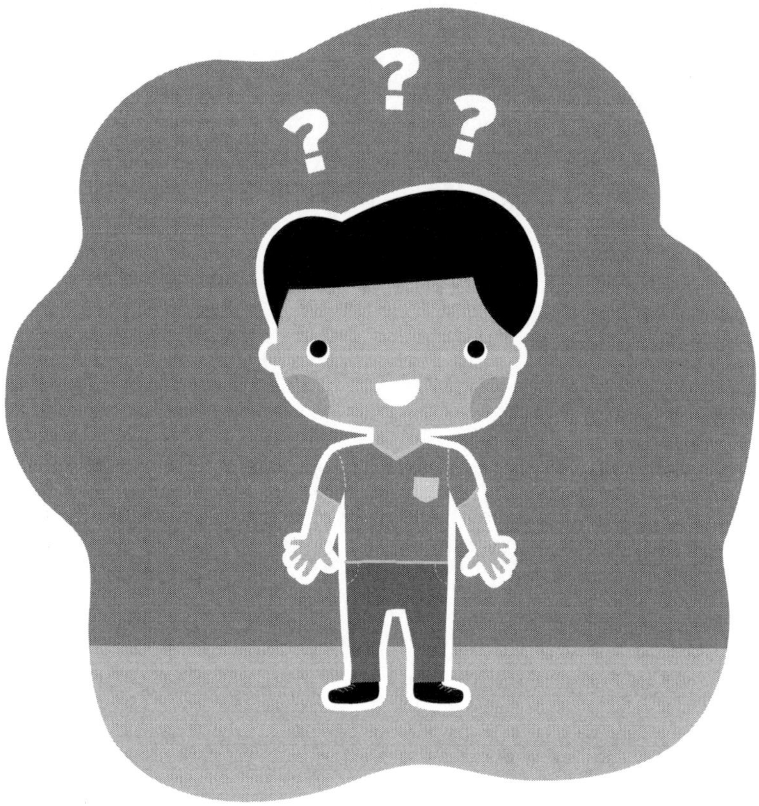

4. **How are twins made?**
   Twins are made in two ways: The first, Fraternal Twins, occur when two eggs get fertilized by two sperm at the same time. These twins don't look exactly alike and can be a boy and a girl. The second, Identical Twins, occur when an egg gets fertilized by one sperm but soon after the baby starts to develop it splits into two. These twins look exactly alike and can only be two boys or two girls.

5. **Do twins each have their own umbilical cords?**
   Yes. Each twin has it's own umbilical cord running from it's belly button to the wall of the womb.

6. **What if a baby comes out too early or too late?**
   When a baby is born too early, the doctor can usually ensure it has everything it needs to continue developing outside the womb. If a baby remains in the womb more than two weeks past it's due date, the doctor will give the woman medicine that starts the birth process.

7. What if the cord gets wrapped around the baby's neck/head?

When this happens, the doctor can usually tell that the baby is in distress (even though it's still in the womb) and can decide whether they need to perform an emergency Cesarean birth in order to untangle the cord quickly. In most cases, the baby is just fine.

8. Does it hurt to have a baby?

Most mums would say that it's a lot of work and sometimes painful, but luckily their bodies forget the pain pretty quickly.

9. How long does it take the baby to grow in the uterus/womb?

It takes approximately forty weeks (nine months) for a baby to grow in the uterus.

10. What if the baby is blue when it's born?

The doctor/midwife can give the baby some oxygen in order to help it breath.

11. What if the baby comes out feet first?

This is called being born in a breech position. The doctor/midwife knows when the baby is in this position (even though it is still in the uterus) and can decide whether they need to perform an emergency Cesarean birth.

12. Does it hurt to have sex?

Sex is supposed to feel good. Our bodies are designed that way so that people will want to reproduce.

13. How long does it take to make a baby?

It only takes a few minutes for the sperm to reach the egg.

14. Can a boy have a baby?

Usually women have the baby because they have the womb where it grows.

15. Do you have to be married to have sex?

You can physically have sex whether you are married or not, but whether or not this is okay depends upon a family's particular values and beliefs.

16. How old do you have to be to have sex?

The law says (insert the legal age of consent for your region). But most adults agree that a person of this age would find it difficult to manage all the responsibilities and consequences that come with having a sexual relationship.

17. Why does the baby come out of the vagina?

The vagina is directly below the womb (where the baby develops) and is designed to stretch in order to let the baby get out through it.

18. How big is the baby when it's born?

Most babies weigh approximately eight pounds when they're born, although some can be bigger or smaller.

19. Do you have to have sex each time you want a baby?

Yes, unless more than one egg is fertilized by sperm at the same time, as in the case of twins, triplets etc.

20. How do you know you're going to have a baby?

A woman can find out if she's pregnant by taking a test from the drug store. If the test is positive, she will usually follow it with a confirmation test done by the doctor.

21. How do you know whether a baby is a boy or a girl?

The doctor can do a test called an ultrasound, which allows them to see the baby's genitals, revealing whether it's a boy or a girl.

22. What makes the baby a boy or a girl?

It's the type of sperm that fertilizes the egg, which determines whether the baby will be a boy or girl.

23. Why do babies sometimes die in the uterus?

This is called a miscarriage and we don't always know why it happens. But we do know that it's the way a woman's body communicates that it isn't feeling healthy enough to carry a baby at that time.

24. How do babies get milk from the breasts?

There are tiny holes in the nipples (the dark areas at the centre of the breasts) through which a baby receives milk.

25. What is sex?

Sex is when a man's penis goes into a woman's vagina. Sex is also a way to describe whether a person is of male or female gender

26. How does the sperm fertilize the egg?

The healthiest and fastest sperm reaches the eggs first, where it breaks down the outer layer of the egg, thereby fertilizing it.

27. How is the egg made?

Every month, natural chemicals in the body called hormones make eggs during a woman's practice pregnancy cycle. Girls are born with about 300,000 of them!

28. Is sperm a seed?

Sperm is commonly referred to as a seed but more accurately, it's a small cell.

29. How is the egg made into a baby?

When the sperm fertilizes the egg, it creates something called DNA, which is like a set of directions for how the baby should develop.

30. How do the sperm and the egg meet?

The sperm swims to the egg and they usually meet in the fallopian tube.

31. Apart from sex, is there any other way to make a baby?

Yes, there are many different ways that doctors can help people become parents. Adults can also adopt babies and children.

32. How does the penis get into the vagina?

When the penis is ready to deliver sperm, it becomes hard (erect), which makes it able to enter the vagina very easily.

33. How long does the penis need to stay in the vagina?

Usually, the penis only needs to stay in the vagina for a few minutes but sometimes this process takes longer, depending on how ready the man's body is to deliver the sperm.

34. Do people lie down to have sex?

Sometimes, but there are many different ways adults can position their bodies to have sex.

35. Where do people have sex?

Usually, sex occurs in the bedroom or somewhere else that is private.

36. How many times do you need to have sex to have a baby?

You only need to have sex once in order to make a baby, but women don't always get pregnant immediately. Sometimes, a man and a woman must have sex several times before they manage to conceive.

37. How do you breathe when you kiss?

You can breathe through your nose when kissing.

38. How old do you have to be to have a baby?

Most girls' bodies are capable of reproducing by about twelve or thirteen years old. But most adults would agree that a child this age would not be ready to be a parent. Different cultures have different rules.

39. Do men have periods?

No. Men don't have eggs or a womb so they can't menstruate. Instead, boys get wet dreams. This is when a small amount of sperm comes out of the penis during sleep, as the testicles begin practicing for creating a baby.

40. How do you know which hole to put the tampon into?

It takes some practice, but girls learn pretty quickly which opening is the vagina. Putting a tampon into the urethra or in the anus wouldn't feel very comfortable.

41. What is puberty?

Puberty is the period in a young person's life (age 8-18) when their child body gradually changes into an adult body. Everyone in the world goes through this process.

42. What makes puberty happen?

Puberty is the result of natural chemicals in the body called hormones.

43. What is a period?

A period is a healthy, normal process that happens when a girl's body is practicing for reproduction. Each month, her uterus grows a lining and when she doesn't get pregnant, this lining leaves the uterus via the vagina in the form of drips. These drips look like blood but they're actually mostly water and tiny bits of skin. Most periods occur monthly and the drips last for about a week at a time.

44. Why are testicles outside the body?

Sperm need to be kept cooler than body temperature so keeping the testicles outside the body ensures that the sperm don't get too warm.

45. Can men have babies?

Usually women have the baby because they have the womb in which it grows.

46. Why do some penises look different?

Boys are born with a loose piece of skin at the end of the penis called a foreskin. Because of particular beliefs or values, some parents decide to have this foreskin removed soon after a boy is born. Although penises often look different, they're all as functional and healthy as each other.

47. What is an erection?

An erection is when a penis becomes hard due to a rush of blood into its spongy tissue. Boys have practice erections several times a day. It's a healthy sign that they're getting ready to have babies someday.

48. What is a condom?

Sometimes adults just want to have sex to show their love for one another, not to make a baby. A condom is a thin rubber sheath that catches sperm during sex, greatly reducing their chances of conceiving. Condoms are clean and healthy when bought from a store but have germs on them after being used so they mustn't be picked up if found.

49. Do you have to be married to have a baby?

No. Many families have parents who are not married. The shape of each wonderful family depends upon their particular values and beliefs.

50. Why are boys' and girls' bodies different?

We're designed differently so that we can reproduce, since both eggs and sperm are needed to make a baby.

51. Why are boys' sex organs on the outside and girls' sex organs on the inside?

In the same way that testicles need to be outside the body to ensure that the sperm stays cooler than body temperature, ovaries need to be inside the body so that eggs can say warm.

9 Quick Answers for Parents:

1. At what age should I initiate conversations about sex with my child?

By the time your child is in preschool, you should be introducing them to basic anatomy/reproduction information, using scientific terms for body parts.

2. My child wants me to tell their friend where babies come from because her mother won't.

It's never appropriate to provide unsolicited sexual education to children other than your own. If you're concerned, approach the parent, stressing to them the importance of sex education as a safety issue.

3. **Won't talking to my child about sex only encourage them to become sexually active?**
   No. Studies show that it's curiosity and ignorance, not knowledge and awareness that lead to early sexual activity.

4. **How much information is too much?**
   It's impossible to give your child too much information. If they're not ready to process something, they quite simply will not.

5. **At what age will my child begin feeling uncomfortable being naked in front of me or uncomfortable seeing me naked?**
   Modesty develops differently in every child. Comfort levels and boundaries (not age) should dictate the timeline for this process. If a child or parent grow uncomfortable being naked in front of family members, that's when it should stop.

6. **Is it appropriate for my child to masturbate?**
   Yes. Masturbation is normal and healthy, providing it occurs in private.

7. **Is it appropriate for my six year-old to play Doctor?**
   No. Although playing doctor is an expression of natural curiosity, it's not appropriate to explore someone else's body. This education should come from a parent with aides such as books, apps and diagrams.

8. **My six year-old walked in on my partner and I having sex. What should I have done?**
   Should this happen to you, calmly asked your child to leave, explaining that you will meet them in their bedroom shortly. If you're comfortable, acknowledge that you and your partner were having sex. If you're not, explain that you were having some private time showing your love for one another and that no one was being hurt.

9. **What if my child says something like, Yuck, those two men are holding hands?**
   Explain that there's nothing wrong with two men holding hands just like there's nothing wrong with a man and a woman holding hands. Reinforce the beauty of diversity and the importance of showing respect for all relationships.

We hope you've enjoyed your journey through **Sex Education: Curiosity Is Getting Complicated!** We welcome your feedback and would love to know what you think. Please take the time to rate us, leave a comment or contact us directly at: **mail@birdeesapp.com**

If you're wondering what's in store for you as your child enters the Elementary School years, we've outlined what you can expect next...

WHAT TO EXPECT NEXT

Parenting becomes more challenging as children's brains and bodies develop towards adulthood.

Here's what you can expect from children ages 9-12:

Change

- *their bodies are transitioning and puberty and growth are at the forefront*
- *experience awkwardness/self consciousness about their bodies*
- *increasing curiosity about sex and sexuality*
- *experience new feelings along with hormonal and physical changes their bodies are undergoing*
- *interaction with a larger social circle (including social networking)*
- *start to feel the influence of peer pressure*
- *push limits as they establish their place in their changing world.*

What do children ages 9-12 need?

Support & Guidance

- *preparation for the road that lies ahead and the many changes that will come with adolescence*
- *reassurance that the physical and emotional changes that come with puberty are normal and everybody goes through them in the transition to adulthood*
- *understanding how their bodies work and how best to care for them*
- *dealing with the many emotional changes that come with adolescence*
- *learning judgment skills and making good decisions*
- *understanding boundaries and respecting family values*
- *accepting responsibility for their actions*
- *knowing when and how to be assertive*
- *developing healthy self esteem and body image*
- *understanding and managing the influence of media and technology*

Sex Education: The Questions Just Got Tougher! outlines the information that you should convey to your child as they grow through the ages of 9 to 12 and will be available for purchase soon. It includes strategies for answering questions, and resources to assist their implementation. Visit us at: www.birdeesapp.com

WHAT'S THAT?

Anus: the opening at the end of our digestive tract (between our buttocks) where stool/solid waste exits the body

Bisexual: someone that is physically/sexually attracted to members of both the same and opposite sex

Bladder: the balloon-like part of the urinary system where urine is stored before is exits the body through the urethra

Breasts: glandular organs situated on the upper chest that are more developed in woman and are used to secrete milk after childbirth to feed the newborn baby

Circumcision: the surgical removal of the foreskin (fold of skin) that covers the tip of the penis

Clitoris: a tiny knob about as big as the end of a little finger that sits above the vulva (labia)

Condom: a thin sheath usually made of rubber that is worn on the penis in men and in the vagina in woman that acts as a barrier to prevent unwanted pregnancies or to provide protection from sexually transmitted infections

Empathy: being able to understand what someone else may be thinking, feeling or experiencing

Erection(s): when a penis becomes hard and stands away from the body, due to a rush of blood into its spongy tissue

Fallopian Tubes: the tube-like part of a woman's reproductive organs that transports the ova (eggs) from the ovaries toward the uterus

Foreskin: a retractable fold of skin that covers the glans(tip) of the penis

Fraternal Twins: twins that are made when two eggs are fertilized by two sperm at the same time

Gay: a term used to describe a homosexual man or woman

Gender: a person's own sense of being either male or female

Gender Identity: a person's own view of being male, female, both or neither

Gender Variant: a person that doesn't conform to being male or female

Genitals: internal and external male and female sex organs involved in reproduction

Heterosexual: someone that is physically/sexually attracted to members of the opposite sex

Homosexual: someone that is physically/sexually attracted to members of the same sex

Identical (Monozygotic) Twins: twins that are made when an egg is fertilized by one sperm but soon after the baby starts to develop it splits into two

Lesbian: a woman that is physically / sexually attracted to other women

Masturbation: touching one's own body and genitals for sexual pleasure

Menarche: the first menstrual bleeding that a female experiences

Menstruation/Period: monthly shedding of the lining of the uterus that moves out of the uterus through the cervix and comes out of the vagina as menstrual blood drops that lasts from 3-5 days

Nocturnal Emissions/Wet Dreams: sexual arousal experienced during sleep that usually results in ejaculation in boys and a feeling of vaginal lubrication in girls

Ovary(ies): the female sex organs that produce ova(um) (eggs)

Penis: the part of the external male sex organ that is designed to deliver sperm into the vagina

Pregnant: carrying a developing baby inside the womb

Private: belonging to that person and not intended for public display or other people

Privates or Private Parts: the genitals, breasts, and mouth

Puberty: the period in a young person's life (age 8-18) when their child body gradually changes into an adult body

Queer: a man who is physically / sexually attracted to other men

Scrotum: an elastic protective pouch of skin that surrounds the testicles.

Sex: a way to describe whether a person is of male or female based on their external genitals

Sex/Intercourse: the act of the penis penetrating the vagina, or any consensual behaviour between two or more individuals of the same or opposite sex involving genital contact and bodily penetration

Sex Organs: the parts of the body that are involved in reproduction and that distinguish us as being male or female based on those organs

Sexual: relating to sex

Sexual Deviancy: abnormal sexual behaviour

Sexual Diversity: issues relating to sexual orientation and gender identity

Sexual Orientation: the emotional, romantic or physical attraction to people of the same, opposite, both, or neither gender

Sexuality: the way people express themselves as sexual beings or the awareness of being either males or female or the way someone is physically attracted to other people

Shame(ful): the feeling that you've done something wrong that needs to be covered up or hidden away from others

Smegma: a secretion (white cheesy substance) from the genitals that collects between the labial folds in females and foreskin of males
Sperm: the male seed or reproductive cell
Stool: the solid waste produced by the digestive system
Testicles (Testes): male sex organs that produce sperm/seed
Testosterone: a male hormone produced by the testicles, that is responsible for growth and sexual development
Transgendered: an individual who identifies with or relates to a gender different to the one that was present at birth
Transsexual: an individual who identifies psychologically with a gender opposite to that of their assigned sex at birth to the point that they want to surgically change their sex
Twins: two babies that are conceived and born at the same time
Urethra: the tube that carries urine from the bladder out of the body through the penis in men and the urethral opening in women
Urine: liquid waste produced by the urinary system that comes out of the body through the urethra
Uterus (Womb): a muscular sac-like organ that houses the developing fetus until birth
Vagina: a tube-like passageway connecting the labia (external genitalia) to the uterus (womb), which acts as a sheath for the penis during intercourse and expands to allow the baby to pass through it during childbirth
Vulva (Labia): the inner (minora) and outer (majora) folds of skin surrounding the vaginal opening
Zygote: the cell made when a male sperm and female egg join, the earliest developmental stage of the embryo

References and Resources

Websites

www.advocatesforyouth.org
www.ashastd.org
www.betterhealth.vic.gov.au
www.birdeesapp.com
www.cfsh.ca
www.crossmap.christianpost.com
www.familieslikemine.com
www.genderspectrum.org
www.goaskalice.columbia.ed
www.guttmacher.org
www.imatyfa.org
www.iwannaknow.org
www.kidshealth.org
www.oprah.com
www.optionsforsexualhealth.org
www.pflag.org
www.pflagcanada.ca
www.planetahead.ca
www.plannedparenthood.org
www.teachingsexualhealth.ca
www.safehealthschools.org
www.sexetc.org
www.sexualityandu.ca
www.sieccan.org
www.siecus.org
www.transactiveonline.org
www.urbandictionary.com

Adult Books

Berman, Dr. Laura. *The Sex Ed Handbook: A Comprehensive Guide for Parents.* Nov. 2012. http://Oprah.com2011

Berkenkamp, Laurie and Steven Atkins. *Talking to your Kids about Sex: A Go Parents! Guide.* Norwich, VT: Nomad Press, 2002.

Brill, Stephanie and Rachel Pepper. *The Transgender Child: A Handbook for Families and Professionals.* San Francisco, CA: Cleis Press Inc, 2008.

Faber, Adele and Elaine Mazlish. *How to Talk So Kids Will Listen & Listen So Kids will Talk.* Updated ed. New York, NY: Scribner, 2012.

Regional Municipality of Halton. Children and Sexuality: *A Guide for Parents and Caregivers of young Children.* www.halton.ca/common/pages/UserFile.aspx?fileId=15448> Halton Region, 2012

Heyman, Richard. *We Need to Talk! Tough Conversations with your Kids: From Sex to Family Values, Tackle Any Topic with Sensitivity and Smarts.* Avon, MA: Adams Media, 2009.

Hickling, Meg. *Boys, Girls and Body Science: A first Book about Facts of Life.* Madeira Park, BC: Harbour Publishing Co. Ltd., 2002.

Hickling, Meg. *The New Speaking of Sex: What Your Children Need to Know and When They Need to Know it.* Kelowna, BC: Northstone, 2005.

Kaeser, Dr. Fred. *What Your Child Needs to Know About Sex (and When): A Straight Talking Guide For Parents.* New York, NY: Celestial Arts, 2011.

Levine, Judith. Harmful to Minors: *The Perils of Protecting Children from Sex.* Minneapolis, MN: University of Minnesota Press, 2002.

Maxwell, Sharon. *The Talk: What Your Kids Need to Hear From YOU About Sex.* Penguin Group (USA) Inc., New York, NY: 2008

Public Health Agency of Canada. *Canadian Guidelines for Sexual Health Education, 2008.* Ottawa, ON: Published by Authority of the Minister of Health, 2008

Public Health Agency of Canada, Minister of Health. *Questions & Answers: Sexual Orientation in Schools.* Published by Authority of the Minister of Health <library.catie.ca/pdf/ATI-20000s/26288E.pdf>.

Rebecca White. *Sex and Relationship Education in Primary School: Professional Development File.* Optimus Professional Publishing Ltd, 2010.

Roffman, Deborah M. *Sex and Sensibility: The Thinking Parent's Guide to Talking Sense About Sex.* Cambridge, MA: Perseus, 2001.

Rosenzweig, Janet.*The Sex-Wise Parent: The Parent's Guide to Protecting Your Child, Strengthening Your Family, and Talking to Kids about Sex, Abuse and Bullying*. New York, NY: Skyhorse Publishing Inc., 2012.

St. Stephen's Community House. *The Little Black Book for Girlz: A Book on Healthy Sexuality.* Toronto, ON: Annick press Ltd., 2008.

St. Stephen's Community House - By Youth for Youth. *The Little Black Book for Guys: Guys Talk About Sex.* Toronto, ON: Annick Press Ltd., 2010.

Sexuality Information and Education Council of the United States. *Guidelines for Comprehensive Sexuality Education: Kindergarten through 12th Grade 3rd ed.* National Guidelines Task Force, 2004. <www2.gsu.edu/guidelines.pdf>

Schwartz, Pepper. *Ten Talks Parents Must Have With Their Children About Sex and Character.* New York, NY: Hyperion, 2000.

Wass, Patricia C. Summer Time - *Sex Education Helps Keep Children Safe from Abuse.* <http://

crossmap.christianpost.com / news / summer-time-sex-education-helps-keep-children-safe-from-abuse-3195> Crossmap, June 2013.

Children's Books

Bourgeois, Paulette and Kim Martyn. *Changes in You and Me: A Book About Puberty, Mostly for Girls, rev ed.* Toronto, ON: Key Porter Books, 2005.

Bourgeois, Paulette & Kim Martyn. *Changes in You and Me: A Book About Puberty, Mostly for Boys, rev ed.* Toronto, ON: Key Porter Books, 2005.

Carr, Jennifer. *Be Who You Are.* Bloomington, IN: Authorhouse, 2010.

Carlson, Nancy. *My family is Forever*. New York: Viking Books, 2004.

Cole, Joanna. *Asking About Sex and Growing Up: A Question-and-Answer Book for Kids.* New York, NY: Harpers Collins, 2009.

Firth, Alex. *What's Happening to Me?* (Boys Edition). London, UK: Usborne Publishing Ltd., 2006.

Harris, Robie H. It's Perfectly Normal: *Changing Bodies, Growing Up, Sex, and Sexual Health.* Cambridge, MA: Candlewick Press, 2009.

Harris, Robie H. *It's so Amazing!: A Book about Eggs, Sperm, Birth, Babies and Families.* Cambridge, MA: Candlewick Press, 2004.

Harris, Robie H. *It's Not the Stork!: A Book about Girls, Boys, Babies, Bodies, Families and Friends.* Cambridge, MA: Candlewick Press, 2008.

Hickling, Meg. *Boys, Girls and Body Science: A first Book about Facts of Life.* Madeira Park, BC: Harbour Publishing Co. Ltd., 2002

Hindman, Jan. A very Touching Book. Ontario, OR: Alexandria Assoc, 1990.

King, Zack and Kimberly King. *I Said No! A Kid-to-Kid Guide to Keeping Private Parts Private.* Weaverville, CA: Boulden, 2010.

Mayle, Peter. *Where did I Come From?* New York, NY: Kensington - Citadel, 1977.

Mayle, Peter. *What's Happening to Me?* New York, NY: Kensington - Citadel, 1981.

Meredith, Susan. *What's happening to me?* (Girls Edition). London, UK: Usborne Publishing Ltd., 2006.

Stones, Rosemary. *Where Do BabiesCome From?* New York, NY: Puffin Books, 1989.

9724870R10047

Printed in Great Britain
by Amazon.co.uk, Ltd.,
Marston Gate.